# Oh's 오지은의 메디컬 영어회화

## .General Hospital

part.1

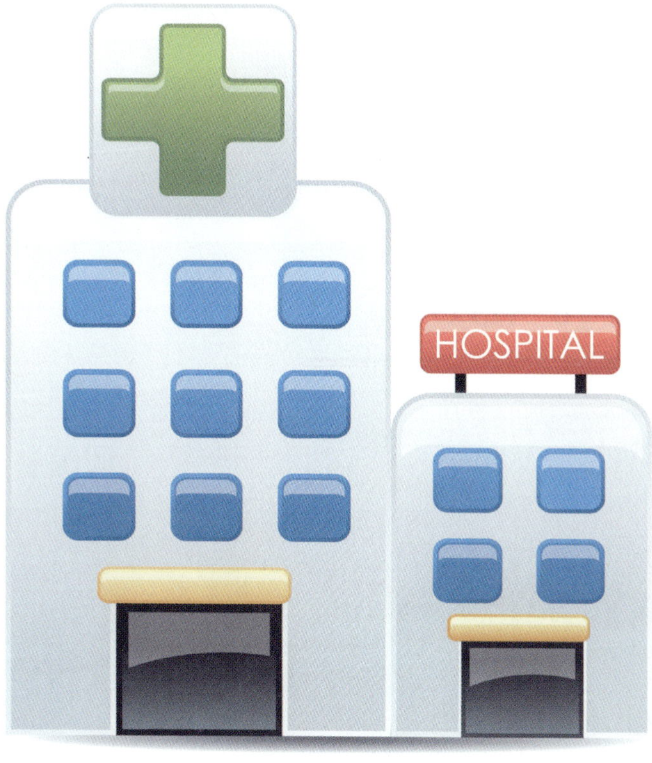


청구문화사

# 오지은의 메디컬 영어회화

2011년 2월 25일 초판인쇄
2011년 3월 10일 초판발행

지은이 / 오지은
펴낸이 / 이상태
펴낸곳 / 청구문화사
120-831 서울특별시 서대문구 연희1동 436-1
전 화 / 02) 332-0541(代)
팩 스 / 02) 337-9577
등 록 / 1990년 11월 2일 제9-247호

ISBN 978-89-5616-433-5 93510

정가 25,000원

## The Story of 오지은의 메디컬 영어회화. General Hospital

오지은의 메디컬 영어회화. General Hospital은 2009년 4월부터 시작하여 2011년 1월 7일에 완성한 저의 첫 번째 메디컬 영어회화책인 종합병원 편입니다.

이 책은 두 가지의 숙제를 풀고 싶은 마음에서 집필하였습니다. 첫 번째 숙제는, 의료 통역이란 난제의 답을 찾는 실마리가 되고 싶었습니다. 의료관광이라는 현장에서 선구자의 역할을 하시는 의료 통역사/의료통역 코디네이터 분들에게 영어권 환자분들의 의료 및 생활 문화와 현지의 살아있는 영어를 알려드리고 싶었습니다. "영어권 환자들은 어디에서 왔는가?" 란 질문에 대한 답을 아실 때 의료통역은 한결 더 수월해지실 것이라 생각됩니다.

두 번째 숙제는 해외에 특히 미국으로 진출하시려는 의료종사자들을 위한 것입니다. 즉 "우리는 어디로 가는가?"에 대한 답을 드리고 싶었습니다. 저는 미국 대학에서 세포병리학을 전공했고 세포병리사로 미국의 병리 연구 산업기관과 지역병원에서 근무를 하였습니다. 아는 만큼 보인다는 격언이 있듯이 십여 년이 넘는 제 미국생활의 경험을 미국의 의료 시장으로 진출을 준비하시고 계시는 분들께 알려드리고 싶었습니다. 미국에 도착 후 가장 먼저 만들어야 하는 Social Security Card를 첫 장에 실은 이유도 여기에 있습니다. 언어는 문화입니다.

그리고 세 번째의 숙제를 추가하자면 아직 재학중인 보건계열 학생 여러분들이 졸업 전에 이 책을 공부하고 졸업 후 내딛는 사회의 첫 발에 도움이 되었으면 합니다. "영어는 권력이다" 라는 말에 저는 한가지를 더 첨가하고 싶습니다. 영어는 "모든 문을 열 수 있는 열쇠이다."

끝으로 저는 오지은의 메디컬영어회화를 수강해주신 모든 수강생님들에게 감사를 전하고 싶습니다. 간호사선생님, 의사선생님, 메디컬코디네이터님, 의료통역사님, 그리고 김천대학교의 물리치료학과 및 의료경영학과 학생들에게 메디컬영어회화를 강의를 하며 만든 책입니다. 현재 의료 현장에 근무하시며 각자의 꿈을 이루기 위해 지금도 저와 같이 향학열을 불태우시며 제게 너무도 소중한 오지은의 메디컬영어회화 1기생 님들이신 송선주 간호사님, 최현경 임상병리사님, 허선희 모발 클리닉 코디네이터님, 김수민 치과코디네이터님들에게 감사를 드립니다. 특히 제게 한국의료문화에 대해 많은 조언을 해주신 순천향대학병원의 간호사 선생님이신 송선주 선생님께 큰 감사를 드립니다. 또한 정동혁 병원경영 컨설턴트님이 제시한 제 책이 지향하는 방향에 대한 사려 깊은 조언에 감사 드리며, 장수경 간호사 선생님, 이비인후과 의사 선생님, 박소영 의료통역사님, 수원의 아주대학병원에서 근무하시는 약사 선생님, 치과 의사 선생님 등 많은 분들이 제 강의를 수강하시며 소중한 자문을 주셨기에 이 책이 세상 밖에 나올 수 있었습니다. 현장의 소리를 담은 책이 되고 싶은 제 꿈을 그 분들이 가능하게 해 주셨습니다.

그리고 메디컬 외국어 회화란 전공과목을 처음으로 한국의 대학교에 개설하신 김천대학교 의료경영학과의 박지원 학과장님과 청구문화사 이상태 대표님께 감사를 드립니다.

이 책의 제목, 표지 디자인 및 다양한 콘텐츠를 이용하실 수 있는
www.ohgieun.com 홈페이지는 B&M Company의 작품입니다. 그들은 천재입니다.
그들에게 무한한 감사의 마음을 전합니다.

## 약력

(현) 오지은의 메디컬 영어회화 연구소장
(현) 이화여자대학교 외국어특수교육대학원 재학 중
(현) 김천대학교 의료경영학과 메디컬 영어회화 외래교수
(현) 연세대학교 원주의과대학 의학영어 외래교수
(현) 강남구 글로벌 헬스케어 코디네이터 회장
성균관대학교-George Town University TESOL자격증

University of Utah 졸업

B.S-Medical Laboratory Sciences Specialization in Cytotechnology
미국 Fortune지 선정 100대 기업, ARUP Air aboratories 근무
미국 Ogden Regional Hospital 근무
미국 세포병리사 면허증, 면허번호 (12697)

**수상 내역:**

Graduation Honored: Cum Laude
University of Utah President's Award
Phi Kappa Phi Honor Society
Phi Eta Sigma Honor Society
Dean's List

## Special Thanks

*Without the Karls, I couldn't finish my first book.*

*I really appreciate all of your help and support.*

*Synghoon Karl*

*Ji-Won Karl*

*Min-Kyu Karl*

*Love,*

*From the bottom of my heart*

## Introduction

Part 1은 외국인 환자분들이 병원내원을 하기 위한 진료예약과 내원 시 첫 접점인 병원 안내데스크 및 진료 후 진료비 수납에 관한 소개로 구성되어 있습니다.

첫 장인 진료예약에서는 외국인 환자분들이 병원내원에 필요한 진료예약을 자택에서 병원으로 하는 전화 진료예약과 병원내원 시 하실 수 있는 검사예약에 대해 소개하였습니다. 또한 병원진료예약 후 진료예약시간의 변경 및 취소에 관한 상황표현과 응급상황 시 병원내원을 위한 응급진료예약도 소개하였습니다. 그리고 진료예약용지(Appointment Reminder)와 병원을 내원하신 외국인 환자분들이 작성해야 하는 문진표(Medical History Form) 양식도 소개하였습니다. 두 양식을 공부하며 실전에 대비하실 수 있도록 연습공간도 만들었습니다.

두 번째 장은 병원 안내데스크입니다. 외국인 환자분들이 병원내원 시 첫 접점인 안내데스크에서 진료실, 각 검사실 및 병원부대시설의 위치안내와 병원진료시간 및 주차시설이용에 관한 문의에 대비하실 수 있도록 많은 표현들을 준비 하였습니다.

세 번째 장은 진료비 수납에 관한 것입니다. 진료비 수납은 의료보험이 있는 외국인 환자와 의료보험이 없는 외국인 환자의 두 가지 상황을 설정하였습니다.예로 해외의료보험에 관한 용어 및 국제의료보험의 양식을 소개하여 직접 작성해보실 수 있도록 하였습니다.

저는 이 책에 미국문화도 간간히 소개하였습니다. 언어는 문화라고 생각합니다. 새로운 언어를 배울 때 그 언어의 문화를 이해하시게 되면 언어 습득에 더 많은 도움이 될 것이라 생각됩니다. 그리하여, 한국의 주민등록증과 유사한 Social Security Card와 미국의 지불방법 중 하나인 개인수표(Personal Check)에 관한 소개 및 직접 작성해 보실 수 있는 작은 공간도 만들었습니다.

Part 1의 진료예약, 병원안내데스크 및 진료비관련 표현은 Part 2는 외국인 환자와 의사선생님과의 진료실 내에서 이루어지는 상황으로 이어집니다.

Part 2는 **Chapter 4: 증상과 징후**, **Chapter 5: 통증** 및 **Chapter 6: 복약지시**로 구성하였습니다. **Part 2** 에서 뵙겠습니다.

# Part 1

## Contents

## Contents

**Contents**

Contents

## Contents

## Chapter 3 Doctor's Fee

## 진료비

## Contents

# Chapter 1

# Making a Doctor's Appointment

# 진료예약하기

## 1. Key Words for Making a Doctor's Appointment
진료예약관련 주요어휘

- **Key Words, 주요어휘**
- ***Code breaker's corner: 로리와 함께 하는 미국문화 엿보기***
    - **Social Security Card, 일종의 미국 주민등록증**

# Key Words

**Appointment,**
**Doctor's Appointment:** 병원예약

**Hospital Hours,**
**Clinic Hours:** 진료시간

**Routine Checkup,**
**General Checkup,**
**Regular Checkup:** 정기검진

**First Visit:** 초진

**Appointment Sheet:** 예약용지

**Examination Slip:** 검사용지

**Referral, Referral Letter:** 의사 소견서

**Registration Form:** 등록용지

**Current Mailing Address:** 현 주소

**Patient Card:** 진료카드

**Medical History Form,**
**New Patient History Form,**
**Health History Form:** 문진표

## *Code breaker's corner: 로리와 함께 하는 미국문화 엿보기*

### Social Security Card: 일종의 미국 주민등록증

모든 서류에 기본적으로 필요한 것이 Social Security 번호 (123-456-7890, 이 카드의 예로는) 입니다. 학교등록, 은행계좌 만들기 등등. 이 번호는 영주권과 상관없이 모든 외국인에게 주어집니다. 미국 시민도 같은 모양의 카드를 소지하고 있습니다. 저도 미국에서 가장 먼저 만든 것이 이 Social Security Card 입니다.

*토익문제에도 자주 등장하는 소재입니다. ☺

For more information, you can visit the web site, **http://www.ssa.gov**

## 2. Telephone Appointment: From your home
전화예약: 자택에서 병원으로 진료예약하기

- **Dialogue, 대화**
- **Words, 어휘**
- **Review, 복습**

# Dialogue

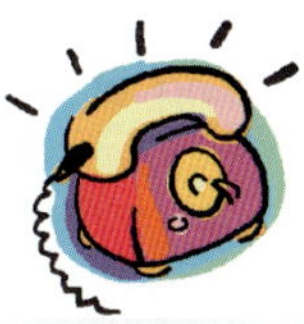

**Receptionist:** Kyung Hee University International Medical Service (**KUIMS**). How may I help you?

**Patient:** I would like to make an appointment to see a doctor.

**Receptionist:** Alright. What is the appointment regarding?

**Patient:** Um. I have been throwing up all day.

**Receptionist:** I see. Have you been here before?

**Patient:** No. This is my first visit.

**Receptionist:** O.K. May I ask your last name please?

**Patient:** Johnson.

**Receptionist:** First name please?

**Patient:** Jeffrey.

**Receptionist:** What's your date of birth?

**Patient:** 11/06/76.

**Receptionist:** What's your day time phone number?

**Patient:** 02-345-6789.

**Receptionist:** Let me check if there are any openings available.

The earliest opening is tomorrow morning at 9:00 a.m.

Will that be a good time for you?

**Patient:** Um, is there an opening at 10 a.m. instead of 9 a.m. on the same day?

**Receptionist:** Well, 10 a.m. is already filled, but there is an opening at 11 a.m. Will that be fine with you?

**Patient:** That's perfect. I will take it.

**Receptionist:** I have you down for 11:00 on Friday morning.

**Patient:** Thank you, ma'am.

**Receptionist:** You're welcome.

If you need to reschedule or cancel your appointment, please give us a call at this number, 02-376-8888, 24 hours in advance.

Is there anything else I can help you with?

**Patient:** Well, nothing else. I really appreciate your help.

Have a nice day!

**Receptionist:** You too, sir.

## Words

* make an appointment to see a doctor: 진료예약을 하다.

* to see a doctor: 진료를 받기 위해

* regarding: 어디가 아프셔서

* throw up: 구토를 하다

* all day: 하루 종일

* first visit: 처음 방문

* last name: 성

* first name: 이름

* date of birth/ Date of Birth (DOB): 생년월일

* openings available: 예약 가능한 시간

* on the same day: 같은 날

* filled: 예약이 되어 자리가 없는

* reschedule: 예약시간을 변경하다

* cancel: 예약을 취소하다.

* in advance: 미리

* appreciate: ~에 감사해하다.

* We have an opening at 3 p.m. = There is an opening at 3 p.m.

**Review:** 각각의 구문을 영작하세요.
정답은 전 페이지의 Dialogue를 참고하세요.

### Telephone Appointment: From your home

**Receptionist:** Kyung Hee University International Medical Service.

How may I help you?

**Patient:** I would like to [진료를 받기 위해 예약을 하다: ]

**Receptionist:** Alright. What is the appointment [어디가 아프셔서: ]

**Patient:** Um. I have been [토하다: ] all day.

**Receptionist:** I see. Have you been here before?

**Patient:** No. This is my [초진: ]

**Receptionist:** O.K. May I ask your [성: ] please?

**Patient:** Johnson.

**Receptionist:** [이름: ] please?

**Patient:** Jeffrey.

**Receptionist:** What's your 생년월일: ?

**Patient:** 11/06/76.

**Receptionist:** What's your

낮 시간에 연락 가능한 전화번호: ?

**Patient:** 02-345-6789.

**Receptionist:** Let me check if there are any

예약 가능한 시간:

가장 이른 예약 가능한 시간은: is

tomorrow morning at 9:00 a.m.

Will that be a good time for you?

**Patient:** Um, is there an opening at 10 a.m. instead of 9 a.m.

같은 날: ?

**Receptionist:** Well, 10 a.m. 이미 예약이 되었습니다:

but there is an opening at 11 a.m.

Will that be fine with you?

**Patient:** That's perfect. 그 시간으로 하겠습니다:

**Receptionist:** I have you down for 11: 00 on Friday morning.

**Patient:** Thank you, ma'am.

**Receptionist:** You're welcome.

If you need to 변경하거나: or 취소:

your appointment, please give us a call at this number, 02-376-8888,

24시간 전에:

Is there anything else I can help you with?

**Patient:** Well, nothing else. 정말 감사합니다:

Have a nice day!

**Receptionist:** You too, sir.

## 3. Key Words for Hospital/Clinic Hours
진료시간관련 주요어휘

- **Key Words, 주요어휘**
- **Drill, 연습문제**
- **Abbreviation for Days of the Week, 각 요일 명 약자 표기**
- **Drill, 연습문제**

Chapter 1

## Key Words

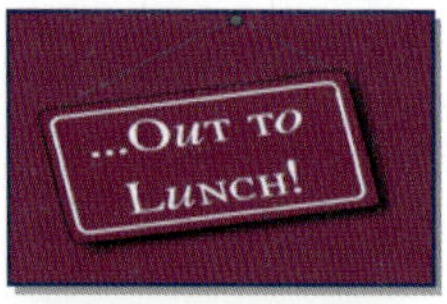


* Closed over lunch hour:
점심시간에는 휴진합니다.

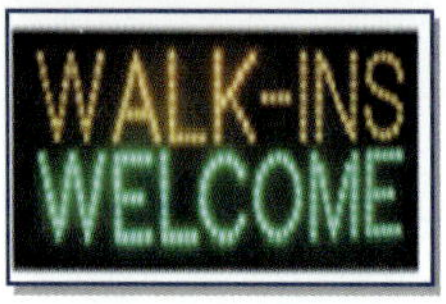


* Walk-ins Welcome: 예약 없이 내원하셔도 환영합니다.
* (=) A drop in basis: 사전 예약 없이 내원 가능.
* Walk-in patient: 예약 없이 내원한 환자.

**Drill: 아래의 진료일정표를 참고하여 문제 1-2에 답하세요.**

**1. 사전 예약없이 내원 가능한 클리닉의 전화번호를 적으세요.**

**2. 점심시간에 휴진하는 클리닉의 주소를 적으세요.**

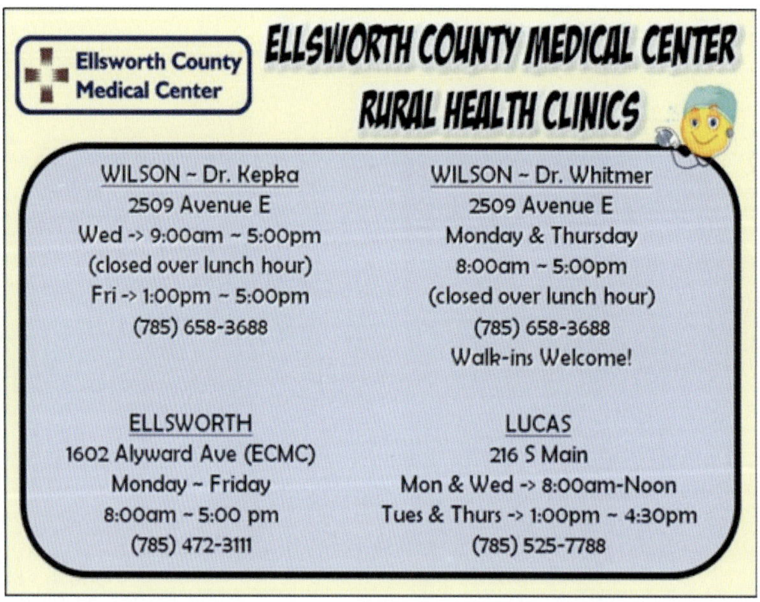

Ellsworth County Medical Center

ELLSWORTH COUNTY MEDICAL CENTER
RURAL HEALTH CLINICS

WILSON ~ Dr. Kepka
2509 Avenue E
Wed -> 9:00am ~ 5:00pm
(closed over lunch hour)
Fri -> 1:00pm ~ 5:00pm
(785) 658-3688

WILSON ~ Dr. Whitmer
2509 Avenue E
Monday & Thursday
8:00am ~ 5:00pm
(closed over lunch hour)
(785) 658-3688
Walk-ins Welcome!

ELLSWORTH
1602 Alyward Ave (ECMC)
Monday ~ Friday
8:00am ~ 5:00 pm
(785) 472-3111

LUCAS
216 S Main
Mon & Wed -> 8:00am-Noon
Tues & Thurs -> 1:00pm ~ 4:30pm
(785) 525-7788

# Abbreviation for Days of the Week

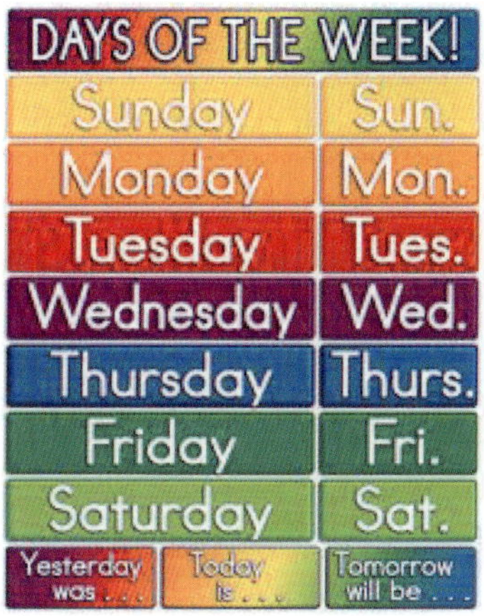


Monday→Mon. → (**M**)
Tuesday→Tues. → (**T**)
Wednesday→Wed. → (**W**)
Thursday→Thurs. → (**Th**)
Friday→Fri. → (**F**)
Saturday→ Sat. → (**S**)
Sunday→ Sun. → (**Su**)

**Drill:** 각 요일의 약자를 기입하세요.

| Day 1 | Day 2 | Day 3 |
|---|---|---|
| Sunday | Monday | Tuesday |
| Sun. | | |
| **Day 4** | **Day 5** | **Day 6** |
| Wednesday | Thursday | Friday |
| | | |
| | **Day 7** | |
| | Saturday | |
| | | |

# 4. Making an Appointment for an MRI exam: At the Doctor's Office

MRI검사예약: 병원에서 검사예약하기

- **Dialogue, 대화**
- **Words, 어휘**
- **Review, 복습**

# Dialogue

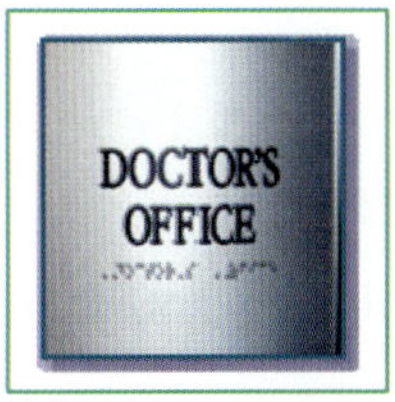


**Patient:** I would like to make an appointment for an MRI exam.

**Doctor's Assistant:** I see. Did your doctor put a STAT order on it?

**Patient:** No, he didn't.

**Doctor's Assistant:** Did you bring a referral from your doctor?

**Patient:** Yes. I brought a referral from my primary care provider for an MRI test.

**Doctor's Assistant:** Could I see your referral please?

**Patient:** Sure. Here you are.

**Doctor's Assistant:** Let me see when we have openings in the schedule. Wait a second please.

**Patient:** O.K.

**Doctor's Assistant:** Today is October $8^{th}$.
Well, sorry we don't have any openings until October $10^{th}$.
The earliest opening is at 9:00 a.m. on October $11^{th}$.
Which day is good for you?

**Patient:** Thursday.

**Doctor's Assistant:** O.K. I'll schedule you for 10:45 a.m. on Thursday, October 11th. Would that be good for you?

**Patient:** Perfect.

**Doctor's Assistant:** I will give you some instructions for the test.

Please have a soft meal for dinner on Wednesday, October 10th and then take this medicine at 8:00 p.m.

After that you need to fast.

**Patient:** All right.

**Doctor's Assistant:** That's all. See you on the exam day.

If you have any questions about this examination, feel free to call us.

There is a phone number at the bottom of the appointment sheet.

**Patient:** Thank you for your help. I'll see you then.

## Words

* STAT order: 긴급한 검사

* STAT: at once, immediately, (의학용어) 긴급한

From a Latin word 'statim' which means immediately

('statim'이란 라틴어로써 '즉시'라는 뜻)

* referral: 소견서

* instructions: 지시사항

* soft meal: 부드러운 음식

* fast: 금식, 금식하다.

* NPO (Nothing Per Mouth): 아무것도 드시지 마세요. 금식하세요.

* feel free to: 언제든지 ~하다.

* at the bottom of: ~의 아래에

* appointment sheet: 예약용지

Chapter 1

**Review:** 각각의 구문을 영작하세요.
정답은 전 페이지의 Dialogue를 참고하세요.

**Patient:** I would like to make an appointment for an MRI exam.

**Doctor's Assistant:** I see. Did your doctor

긴급한 검사라고 하셨나요?:

**Patient:** No, he didn't.

**Doctor's Assistant:** Did you bring a 소견서: from your doctor?

**Patient:** Yes. I brought a 소견서: from my 주치의:

for an MRI test.

**Receptionist:** Could I see your 소견서: please?

**Patient:** Sure. Here you are.

**Doctor's Assistant:** Let me see when we have

예약 가능한 날짜:

Wait a second please.

**Patient:** O.K.

**Doctor's Assistant:** Today is October $8^{th}$.

Well, sorry we don't have any openings **까지:** October $10^{th}$.

The earliest opening is at 9:00 a.m. on October $11^{th}$.

**어느 날이 좋으세요?:**

**Patient:** Thursday.

**Doctor's Assistant:** O.K. I'll **예약해 드리겠습니다:**

10:45 a.m. on Thursday, October $11^{th}$.

Would that be good for you?

**Patient:** Perfect.

**Doctor's Assistant:** I will give you **검사에 필요한 지시사항:**

Please have a **저녁으로 부드러운 음식을:** on

Wednesday, October $10^{th}$ and then take this medicine at 8:00 p.m.

**그 후에는:** you need to **금식:**

**Patient:** All right.

**Doctor's Assistant:** That's all. See you **검사 당일에:**

If you have any questions about this examination,

**언제든지 전화주세요:**

There is a phone number **예약용지 하단에**:

**Patient:** Thank you for your help. I'll see you then.

## 5. Appointment Reminder
진료예약서

- **What is an Appointment Reminder? 진료예약서란?**
- **Review: Filling Out My Appointment Reminder,**

  **나의 진료예약서 작성하기**

# What is an Appointment Reminder?

## Appointment Reminder

**What do I need to bring on the day of my appointment?**

**Please bring these to your appointment:**

- ☐ This appointment sheet
- ☐ Health insurance card
- ☐ Co-pay if needed by your insurance plan
- ☐ A list of the medicines, vitamins and herbs you take

**Copies of:**

- ☐ X-rays
- ☐ lab tests
- ☐ medical records

**Your Appointment:**

Patient's Name ______________________________________

Your ____________________________________________ is on
(Test or Surgery)

☐ Monday ☐ Tuesday ☐ Wednesday ☐ Thursday ☐ Friday
☐ Saturday ☐ Sunday

__________ _____ 20________ at ________________
Month Date Year Time

Location/Building ______________________________________

Address______________________________________________

Clinic/Doctor __________________Telephone _______________

Please check in at the registration desk ____ minutes before your appointment.

If you are not able to keep this appointment, please call____________.

## Review: Filling Out My Appointment Reminder

본인의 진료예약서를 작성하면서 주요단어와 구문을 익혀보는 공간입니다.

Part 1의 정답은 전 페이지를 참고 하세요.

Part 2의 정답은 정답 및 해석부분에 있습니다.

### Part 1

진료예약서:

**What do I need to bring**
예약 당일에:

**Please bring these to your appointment:**

- ☐ 이 진료예약서:
- ☐ 의료보험 카드:
- ☐ 공동부담액: if needed by your insurance plan

☐ A list of the 약: , vitamins and 한약: you take

사본:

- ☐ 엑스레이 결과:
- ☐ 검사 결과:
- ☐ 진료 기록:

## Part 2

### Your Appointment:

Patient's Name

______________________________________________

Your ____________________________________________ is on

(Test or Surgery)

☐ Monday ☐ Tuesday ☐ Wednesday ☐ Thursday ☐ Friday

☐ Saturday ☐ Sunday

| ____________ | _____ | 20_______ | at __________ |
|---|---|---|---|
| Month | Date | Year | Time |

Location/Building ________________________________________

Address _____________________________________________

Clinic/Doctor ______________________ Telephone ______________

Please 접수하세요: at the registration desk ____ minutes before your appointment.

If you are not able to keep this appointment, please call________________.

## 6. Telephone Appointment: Cancellation
전화예약: 진료예약 취소

- **Dialogue, 대화**
- **Words, 어휘**
- **Review, 복습**

Chapter 1

# Dialogue

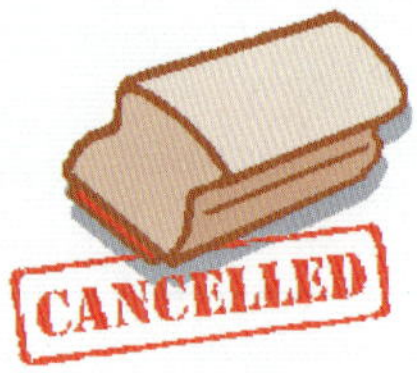


**Receptionist:** Accurate Medical Imaging Radiology Center. What can I do for you this morning?

**Patient:** I would like to cancel my appointment.

**Receptionist:** Alright. What's your last name please?

**Patient:** Johnson.

**Receptionist:** First name please?

**Patient:** Jeffrey.

**Receptionist:** And your date of birth, please?

**Patient:** 11/06/76.

**Receptionist:** You have an appointment with us at 3 o'clock on March $7^{th}$.

**Patient:** That's correct, ma'am. I have an urgent business trip on the same day, so I need to cancel it please.

**Receptionist:** I see. I will cancel it for you.
When you come back from your trip, please give us a call for your new appointment. Have a nice business trip, sir.

**Patient:** Thank you. I really appreciate all your help.
Have a nice day.

## Words

* cancel: ~을 취소하다

* urgent: 급한

* business trip: 출장

* on the same day: 같은 날에

* give us a call: 우리에게 전화해 주세요.

* 상대방이 여성일 경우 ma'am을 사용함

* 상대방이 남성일 경우 sir을 사용함

## Review: 각각의 구문을 영작하세요.

정답은 전 페이지의 Dialogue를 참고하세요.

**Telephone Appointment: Cancellation**

**Receptionist:** Accurate Medical Imaging Radiology Center.

What can I do for you this morning?

**Patient:** I would like to [예약을 취소하고 싶습니다:]

**Receptionist:** Alright. What's your last name please?

**Patient:** Johnson.

**Receptionist:** First name please?

**Patient:** Jeffrey.

**Receptionist:** And your date of birth, please?

**Patient:** 11/06/76.

**Receptionist:** You [저희 병원에 예약이 되셨군요:] at

3 o'clock on March 7th.

**Patient:** That's correct, ma'am.

급한 출장을 가야 합니다: on the same day, so I need to cancel it please.

**Receptionist:** I see. I will cancel it for you.

출장 다녀오신 후: , please give us a call for your new appointment. Have a nice business trip, sir.

**Patient:** I really appreciate all your help.

Have a nice day.

## 7. Medical History Form
문진표

- What is a Medical History Form? 문진표란?
- Words, 어휘
- Review: Filling Out My Medical History Form,
  복습: 나의 문진표 작성하기

# What is a Medical History Form?

**Medical History Form**

Name ______________________________________________

Date of Birth ________________________

Sex ______ Age _____

What is the present state of your general health?

__________________________________________

Physician's Name _______________ Phone _________________

What medications are you presently taking?

_____________________________________________

Are you now or have you been pregnant within the past three months? ______________________

Has your physician restricted your participation in exercise?

_______________________________

If yes, please describe

__________________________________________________

**Do you have now or have you ever had? Yes No**

1. A history of heart problems? _____ _____

2. A history of lung disease? _____ _____

3. Chest, neck, and/or jaw pains/discomforts at rest or during exertion? _____ _____

4. Difficulty with physical exercise, such as chest pain/discomfort, dizziness or extreme shortness of breath? _____ _____

5. Muscle, joint, or back disorder that could be aggravated by physical activity? _____ _____

If yes, please describe ______________________________

6. A chronic illness? _____ _____

If yes, please list __________________________________

7. High blood pressure? _____ _____

8. Diabetes? _____ _____

9. Cigarette-smoking habit? _____ _____

10. High blood cholesterol? _____ _____

11. History of heart problems in a 1st degree relative (parents, siblings, children)? _____ _____

If yes, at what age?

Mother _____ Father _____ Brother _____ Sister _____

Son _____ Daughter _____

12. Would you describe your lifestyle as sedentary? (No regular exercise or active recreational pursuits)? _____ _____

If no, please describe your exercise program

________________________________________

13. Are you a male over age 45 or a female over age 55?

_____ _____

To the best of my knowledge, the above information is accurate and complete.

Signature ________________________________________

Date ____________________

Chapter 1

## Words

* exertion: 힘든 일(운동)

* disorder: 질환

* dizziness: 어지러움

* extreme shortness of breath: 극심하게 숨이 차는 것

* aggravate: 악화되다

* chronic illness: 만성질환

* High blood pressure: 고혈압

* Diabetes: 당뇨병

* High blood cholesterol: 고지혈증

* 1st degree relative: 직계가족

* siblings: 형제자매

* sedentary: 활동적이지 못한

## Review: Filling Out My Medical History Form

본인의 문진표를 작성하면서 주요단어와 구문을 익혀보는 공간입니다.

**Let me fill it out and bring it back to you!**

Name ______________________________________________

Date of Birth _________________________

Sex ______ Age _____

What is the present state of your general health?

__________________________________________

Physician's Name ________________ Phone __________________

What medications are you presently taking?

_____________________________________________

Are you now or have you been pregnant within the past three months?

______________________

Has your physician restricted your participation in exercise?

_______________________________

If yes, please describe

__________________________________________________

**Do you have now or have you ever had? Yes No**

1. A history of heart problems? _____ ____

2. A history of lung disease? _____ ____

3. Chest, neck, and/or jaw pains/discomforts at rest or during exertion? _____ ____

4. Difficulty with physical exercise, such as chest pain/discomfort, dizziness or extreme shortness of breath? _____ ____

5. Muscle, joint, or back disorder that could be aggravated by physical activity? _____ ____

If yes, please describe ________________________________

6. A chronic illness? _____ ____

If yes, please list ________________________________

7. High blood pressure? _____ ____

8. Diabetes? _____ ____

9. Cigarette-smoking habit? _____ ___

10. High blood cholesterol? _____ ___

11. History of heart problems in a 1st degree relative (parents, siblings, children)? _____ ___

If yes, at what age?

Mother _____ Father _____ Brother _____ Sister _____

Son _____ Daughter _____

12. Would you describe your lifestyle as sedentary? (No regular exercise or active recreational pursuits)? _____ ___

If no, please describe your exercise program

________________________________________

13. Are you a male over age 45 or a female over age 55? _____ ___

To the best of my knowledge, the above information is accurate and complete.

Signature ________________________________________

## 8. Telephone Appointment: Reschedule
전화예약: 진료예약 재 조정하기

- **Dialogue, 대화**
- **Words, 어휘**
- **Review, 복습**

# Dialogue

**Receptionist:** Accurate Medical Imaging Service Center.

Good morning, ma'am. What can I do for you this morning?

**Patient:** I have an MRI exam on November $10^{th}$ at 9 a.m., but I don't think I can do my MRI exam on that day. Can I reschedule it at 2 o'clock in the afternoon on November $3^{rd}$ if it's possible, please?

**Receptionist:** Let me check if there are any openings available on that day.

Thank you for waiting.

I am afraid we don't have any openings till 3:00 p.m., unless there is a cancellation.

**Patient:** Well, I can take MRI any time after 3:00.

**Receptionist:** Good then. We have an opening at 3:30.

Can you take it instead?

**Patient:** Wow. I will take it. It couldn't be better.

**Receptionist:** Let me double make sure.

Your new appointment is on November $3^{rd}$ at 3:30.

**Patient:** That's correct.

Thank you very much. I really appreciate that.

Have a good one. Bye.

**Receptionist:** You too, Bye.

**Chapter 1**

---

## Words

* on that day: 그날

* reschedule: 예약을 다시 하다

* I am afraid: 죄송하지만

* It couldn't be better: 가장 좋다

* double make sure: 다시 확인하겠습니다

**Review:** 각각의 구문을 영작하세요.
정답은 전 페이지의 Dialogue를 참고하세요.

**Telephone Appointment: Reschedule**

**Receptionist**: Accurate Medical Imaging Service Center.

Good morning, ma'am. What can I do for you this morning?

**Patient:** I have an MRI exam on November 10th at 9 a.m., but [MRI 검사를 받을 수 없을 것 같습니다:] on that day.

Can I [예약을 다시 하다:] at 2 o'clock in the afternoon on November 3rd [만일 가능하다면:] please?

**Receptionist:** Let me check if there are [예약 가능한 시간:] on that day. Thank you for waiting.

I am afraid we don't have any openings [까지:] 3:00 p.m., [취소되지 않는 한:]

**Patient:** Well, [저는 MRI검사를 오후 3시 이후에는 언제든지 받을 수 있습니다:]

**Receptionist:** Good then.

3:30에 예약이 가능합니다:

이 시간으로 대신 예약 하시겠습니까?:

**Patient:** Wow. 아주 좋습니다:

그 시간으로 예약 하겠습니다:

**Receptionist:** 다시 확인하겠습니다:

고객님의 새 일정은 11월 3일 오후 3시 30분입니다:

**Patient:** That's correct.

Thank you very much. I really appreciate that.

Have a good one. Bye.

**Receptionist:** You too, Bye.

## 9. Telephone Appointment: Urgent Care
전화예약: 응급상황

- **Dialogue, 대화**
- **Words, 어휘**
- **Review, 복습**

# Dialogue

**Receptionist:** Doctor's office. Linda speaking.

How can I help you?

**Patient:** I need to make an appointment with Dr. Park.

**Receptionist:** Could I have your name, please?

**Patient:** Jeffrey Johnson.

**Receptionist:** Okay, Mr. Johnson.

What do you need to see the doctor about?

**Patient:** Well, I've been suffering from a headache for more than a week, and my headache is getting worse each day. I am running a high fever as well.

**Receptionist:** Hmm. Dr. Park is off tomorrow.

Do you think you can wait until the day after tomorrow?

**Patient:** Oh, I do really hope to get in today.

I can't take it anymore.

Maybe I'll have to go to the walk-in clinic instead.

**Receptionist:** Wait a minute.

We had a cancellation for 3:00 p.m. today.

Do you think you can make it?

**Patient:** I think I can make it if I leave right now.

**Receptionist:** We're running a bit behind schedule, so you can probably count on seeing Dr. Park around three-thirtyish.

**Patient:** That's great. Thanks for fitting me in.

**Receptionist:** No problem, Mr. Johnson.

We'll see you in an hour or so.

**Chapter 1**

---

## Words

* urgent care: 응급상황

* suffering from ~: ~로 고생하고 있다

* each day: 매일

* running a high fever: 고열이 있다

* the day after tomorrow: 모레

* get in: 진료를 보다

* walk-in clinic: 예약 없이 진료를 받을 수 있는 클리닉

* I can make it: 제 시간에 도착할 수 있을 것 같습니다.

* a bit: 조금

* behind schedule: 예정보다 지연되다, 밀리다

* three-thirtyish: 세시 삼십 분경, 대략 세시 삼십 분대

* an hour or so: 한 시간 가량

**Review:** 각각의 구문을 영작하세요.
**정답은 전 페이지의 Dialogue를 참고하세요.**

**Telephone Appointment: Urgent care**

**Receptionist:** Doctor's office. Linda speaking.

How can I help you?

**Patient:** 박선생님에게 진료를 보려고 예약을 하고

싶습니다:

**Receptionist:** Could I have your name, please?

**Patient:** Jeffrey Johnson.

**Receptionist:** Okay, Mr. Johnson.

What do you need to see the doctor about?

**Patient:** Well, I've been 두통으로 고생하고 있습니다: for

more than a week, and

매일 두통이 심해지고 있습니다: .

I am 고열도 있습니다: as well.

**Receptionist:** Hmm. Dr. Park 내일 휴진입니다:

Do you think you can wait until the day after tomorrow?

**Patient:** Oh, I do really hope to 오늘 꼭 진료를 보고 싶습니다:

I can't take it anymore.

Maybe I'll have to go to 예약 없이 진료를 받을 수 있는 클리닉:

instead.

**Receptionist:** Wait a minute.

We had a 오늘 3시 예약이 취소 되었습니다:

그 시간에 내원하실 수 있겠습니까?:

**Patient:** I think I can make it if I leave right now.

**Receptionist:** We're 진료가 예정보다 조금 밀립니다: ,

so you can probably

박선생님에게 진료를 보실 수 있을 겁니다:

around 세시 삼십 분경:

**Patient:** That's great.

| 그 시간으로 예약해 주셔서 감사합니다: |
|---|

**Receptionist:** No problem, Mr. Johnson.

We'll see you | 약 한 시간 후: |

## 10. Key Expressions for Making a Doctor's Appointment
진료예약 관련 주요구문

- Drill, 각 상황별 진료예약표현 연습문제

  - 진료예약없이 내원을 할 경우
  - 진료예약을 할 수 없을 경우
  - 의사선생님의 진료시간에 관련된 질문사항
  - 진료예약 가능한 시간/요일에 관련된 질문
  - 진료예약을 취소할 경우
  - 병원/클리닉 진료시간 관련 질문
  - 진료예약시간 확인
  - 기타

**Drill:** 각 상황별 진료예약 표현을 영작 하세요.

## 진료예약없이 내원을 할 경우

1. 예약이 되어 있지는 않은데요, 너무 급합니다.

   ______________________________ , but it's extremely urgent.

2. 예약 없이 내원해도 됩니까?

   ______________________________without a scheduled appointment?

Chapter 1

## 진료예약을 할 수 없을 경우

1. 죄송합니다만, 취소가 없는 한 11시 까지는 빈자리가 없습니다.

   ______________________but we don't have any openings

   till 11:00, ____________________________________

2. 예약일정이 내일 아침까지는 빡빡합니다. 하지만 모레에는 좀

   비어 있습니다.

   Our schedule is ________________________, but there are

   some openings in the schedule ________________________

3. 모레까지 예약이 꽉 찼습니다.

   _____________________________till the day after tomorrow.

4. 이미 예약이 다 찼습니다.

   It's already ___________________

5. 이번 주에는 자리가 없습니다.

   We're ______________________________________________

## 의사선생님의 진료시간에 관련된 질문사항

1. Dr. Park은 12월 16일, 금요일에 진료가 없습니다.

   Dr. Park ____________on Friday, December 16$^{th}$.

   Dr. Park ____________on Friday, December 16$^{th}$.

   * off duty: 휴진

2. Dr. Park은 휴진이십니다. Dr. Joe가 당신의 진료를 보실 것 입니다.

   Dr. Park________________ _______________Dr. Joe.

3. Dr. Joe는 12월 27일과 28일 주말에 진료를 보십니다.

   Dr. Joe _______________________, December 27$^{th}$ and 28$^{th}$.

   * on duty: 진료를 보는

Chapter 1

## 진료예약 가능한 시간/요일에 관련된 질문

1. 현재 제가 예약되어 있는 날짜보다 더 이른 날짜로 예약을 할 수 있을까요?

   Is it possible to make an appointment ____________________

   ________________________________________________________

2. 아침 이른 시간으로 예약을 할 수 있을까요?

   Could I possibly make an appointment for ________________

   ________________________________________________________

3. 11시 이전으로 예약 가능하겠습니까?

   Is it possible to make an appointment for _________________

   ________________________________________________________

4. 어느 시간이 좋으세요?

   ________________________________________________________

5. 2시 45분 예약은 어떻습니까?

   Would 2:45 be ______________________

   How about 2:45?

   How does __________________________

6. 죄송하게도 오늘은 불가능하고 가장 빠른 시간은 내일 아침 9시입니다.

   I am afraid that ______________________________

   ______________________ is tomorrow morning at 9:00 a.m.

7. 어느 날이 좋으세요?

   ______________________________

8. 15일 목요일로 예약 해 드릴까요?

   Can I ______________________________

9. 2월 3일 괜찮으시겠습니까?

   ______________________________

10. 가능하면 빨리 진찰을 받고 싶군요.

    I'd like to see a doctor ______________________

11. 잠깐만. 예약이 가능한지 보겠습니다.

    Just a second, please.

    Let me see______________________________

## 진료예약을 취소할 경우

1. 스케줄을 다시 잡기를 원하거나 취소를 원하시면 우리에게 연락을 주십시오. 전화번호는 290-6085입니다.

   If you want to ______________________________, please give us a call.
   The phone number is 290-6085.

2. 만일 사정이 생겨서 예약시간에 내원하지 못한다면, 적어도 24시간 전에는 알려주세요.

   If for any reason you are unable to make your scheduled appointment, ______________________________________

3. 예약한 날짜에 가지 못하면 어떻게 해야 하지요?

   ______________________________________________________

## 병원/클리닉 진료시간 관련 질문

1. 병원/클리닉 진료시간을 알려 주시겠습니까?

   What are ________________________________________

   ________________________________________clinic hours?

   What are ________________________________________

   * What are your business hours? 영업시간이 어떻게 되나요?

   * What are your office hours? 공공기관 등의 시간, 교수님들과 면담 가능한 시간 등을 알고 싶을 때의 표현법.

## 진료예약시간 확인

1. 10시에 진료 예약을 했습니다.

   ______________________________

2. 다음 진료예약일정은 11월 20일입니다.

   Your next appointment is ______________________

## 기타

1. 어디가 아프셔서 예약을 하십니까?

______________________________________________

______________________________________________

2. MRI검사 예약을 하려면 제 주치의 선생님의 소견서가 필요합니까?

________________ from my ________________ to make an appointment for an MRI exam?

* primary care provider: 주치의

3. 치과 정기검진예약을 인터넷으로 할 수 있을까요?

________________________________for my regular dental checkup?

4. 진료일정이 약 한 시간 정도 밀려있습니다.

______________________________________________

5. 예약이 취소되어 빈자리가 생기면 연락 드리겠습니다.

We'll call you ______________________________

## 11. 정답 및 해석

## 2. 전화예약: 자택에서 병원으로 전화예약

**Receptionist:** 강동경희대병원 국제 클리닉센터입니다.

무엇을 도와드릴까요?

**Patient:** 진료를 받기 위해 예약을 하고 싶습니다.

**Receptionist:** 어디가 아프셔서 예약을 하십니까?

**Patient:** 하루 종일 구토를 합니다.

**Receptionist:** 전에 내방하신 적이 있습니까?

**Patient:** 아닙니다. 이번이 처음 방문입니다.

**Receptionist:** 고객님 성이 무엇입니까?

**Patient:** 존슨입니다.

**Receptionist:** 이름은 무엇입니까?

**Patient:** 제프리입니다.

**Receptionist:** 생년월일을 알려주세요.

**Patient:** 1976년 11월 06일 입니다.

**Receptionist:** 낮 시간에 연락 가능한 전화번호를 알려 주세요.

**Patient:** 02-345-6789 입니다.

**Receptionist:** 예약 가능한 시간이 있는지 확인해 보겠습니다.

가장 이른 예약 가능한 시간은 내일 아침 9시입니다.

이 시간이 괜찮습니까?

**Patient:** 음, 같은 날 오전 9시 대신에 오전 10시에 자리가 있나요?

**Receptionist:** 음, 10시에는 이미 예약이 되었으나 11시에는 자리가 있습니다. 이 시간은 괜찮으십니까?

**Patient:** 아주 좋습니다. 그 시간으로 하겠습니다.

**Receptionist:** 고객님의 예약일정은 금요일 오전 11시 입니다.

**Patient:** 감사합니다.

**Receptionist:** 천만에요.

만일 고객님이 예약시간을 변경하거나 또는 예약을 취소하려면, 02-376-8888으로 24시간 전에 미리 연락해 주세요.

제가 또 도와드릴 것이 있습니까?

**Patient:** 없습니다. 정말 감사합니다.

좋은 하루 되세요.

**Receptionist:** 고객님도요.

## 3. 진료시간관련 주요어휘

### 정답

**연습문제**

1. 예약없이 가능한 클리닉 전화번호: (785)658-3688

2. 점심시간에 휴진하는 클리닉의 주소: 2509 Avenue E

**연습문제**

Mon.
Tues.
Wed.
Thurs.
Fri.
Sat.
Sun.

## 4. 전화예약: 병원에서 검사 예약하기

**Patient:** MRI검사를 받기 위해 예약을 하고 싶습니다.

**Doctor's Assistant:** 알겠습니다.

담당의사 선생님이 긴급한 검사라고 하셨나요?

**Patient:** 아닙니다.

**Doctor's Assistant:** 의사선생님의 소견서를 가지고 오셨나요?

**Patient:** 예. 제 주치의로부터 MRI검사를 위한 의사소견서를 받아왔습니다.

**Doctor's Assistant:** 소견서를 볼 수 있을까요?

**Patient**: 물론이죠. 여기요.

**Doctor's Assistant:** 제가 예약 가능한 날짜가 있는지 알아보겠습니다.

잠시만 기다려 주세요.

**Patient:** 네.

**Doctor's Assistant:** 오늘이 10월 8일이지요.

음, 죄송하지만 10월 10일까지 빈 자리가 없네요.

가장 이른 시간이 10월 11일 오전 9시입니다.

어느 날이 좋으세요?

**Patient:** 목요일이요.

**Doctor's Assistant:** 그러면, 제가 10월 11일 목요일 오전 10시 45분으로 예약해 드리겠습니다. 괜찮으시겠습니까?

**Patient**: 아주 좋습니다.

**Doctor's Assistant:** 검사에 필요한 지시사항을 알려 드리겠습니다.

10월 10일 수요일 저녁은 부드러운 음식으로 하세요.

그리고 이 약을 저녁 8시에 드세요.

그 후에는 금식하세요.

**Patient**: 알겠습니다.

**Doctor's Assistant:** 다 되셨습니다 검사 당일에 뵙겠습니다.

만일 이 검사에 관해 질문이 있다면, 언제든지 전화주세요.

예약용지 하단에 전화번호가 있습니다.

**Patient:** 도와주셔서 감사합니다. 그때 뵙겠습니다.

## 5. 진료예약서란?

**진료예약서**

**예약 당일날 무엇을 가지고 와야 하나요:**

**아래 항목들을 갖고 오십시오:**

- □ 이 진료예약서:
- □ 의료보험 카드:
- □ 보험에서 요구되는 경우 공동부담액:
- □ 복용하고 있는 약, 비타민, 한약들의 목록:

**사본:**

- □ 엑스레이 결과:
- □ 검사 결과:
- □ 진료 기록:

**예약 내용:**

환자 이름: ____________________

귀하의 ____________________ 예약 일시:

(검사나 수술)

□ 월요일: □ 화요일: □ 수요일: □ 목요일:

□ 금요일: □ 토요일: □ 일요일:

____________ ____ 20______ __________

월: 일: 연도: 시간:

위치/건물: ____________________

주소: ____________________

병원/의사: ____________ 전화: __________

예약시간 ___ 분 전에 접수처에서 접수하세요.

만약 이 예약 시간을 지킬 수 없으면 ________로 전화하시기 바랍니다.

## 진료예약서

## Part 2 정답

### Part 2

**Your Appointment:**

Patient's Name **Lorri Oh**

Your **Blood Test** is on
(Test or Surgery)

□ Monday □ Tuesday □ Wednesday □ Thursday ✓Friday
□ Saturday □ Sunday

| **03** | **20** | **2011** | at **2:00 p.m.** |
|---|---|---|---|
| Month | Date | Year | Time |

Location/Building **University of Utah Medical Center**

Address **50 N SLC, UT 84125**

Clinic/Doctor **Jason Park** Telephone **02-234-5678**

Please **접수하세요: check in** at the registration desk 30 minutes before your appointment.

If you are not able to keep this appointment, please call **02-910-1112**.

## 6. 전화예약: 진료예약 취소

**Receptionist:** Accurate Medical Imaging Radiology Center 입니다.

무엇을 도와드릴까요?

**Patient:** 예약을 취소하고 싶습니다.

**Receptionist:** 알겠습니다. 성이 무엇입니까?

**Patient:** 존슨입니다.

**Receptionist:** 이름은요?

**Patient:** 제프리입니다.

**Receptionist:** 생년월일은요?

**Patient:** 1976년 11월 06일입니다.

**Receptionist:** 3월7일 오후 3시에 저희 병원에 예약이 되셨군요.

**Patient:** 예, 맞습니다. 예약한 날과 같은 날에 급한 출장을 가야 합니다.

그래서 예약을 취소해야 합니다.

**Receptionist:** 알겠습니다. 예약을 취소해 드리겠습니다.

출장 다녀오신 후, 예약을 다시 잡기 위해 전화해 주세요.

출장 잘 다녀오세요.

**Patient:** 도와 주셔서 정말 감사합니다. 즐거운 하루 되세요.

## 7. 문진표란

**문진표**

성명 ______________________________

생년월일_________________

성별____ 나이 ___

현재 당신의 건강상태는 어떠한가요? _____________________________

주치의 성명 _________________________

전화번호 ____________

현재 무슨 약을 복용하고 계시나요?_______________________________

당신은 현재 임신 중이거나 또는 지난 3개월 내에

임신한 적이 있습니까? _______

주치의가 당신이 운동하는 것을 금했나요? _____________________

만일 금지했다면, 상세히 기술하세요. _______________________________

현재 당신은 아래와 같은 사항에 해당 하거나 또는 경험이 있나요?

예 또는 아니오 로 답하세요.

1. 심장질환 병력? ___ ___

2. 폐질환 병력? ___ ___

3. 휴식을 취하거나 또는 힘든 일(운동)을 하는 도중 흉부, 목 및/또는 턱에 통증/불편함? ____ ____

4. 흉통/불편함, 어지러움 또는 극심하게 숨이 차는 것으로 인한 육체적 운동의 어려움 ____ ____

5. 신체 활동으로 인해 근육, 관절 또는 등 질환이 악화되나요? ____ ____

만일 그러하다면, 상세히 기술하시오. ________________________

6. 만성질환? ____ ____

만일 만성질환이 있다면, 모두 기록하세요. ______________________________

7. 고혈압이 있나요? ____ ____

8. 당뇨병이 있나요? ____ ____

9. 담배를 피우시나요? ____ ____

10. 고지혈증이 있나요? ____ ____

11. 직계가족 (부모님, 형제자매, 아이들)에 심장질환 병력? ____ ____

만일, 직계가족에 심장 병력이 있다면, 몇 살에 발병했나요?

엄마 ____ 아빠 ____ 남자 형제 ____ 여자 형제 ____ 아들 ____ 딸 ____

12. 당신의 생활방식을 활동적이지 않다고 묘사하시겠습니까?

(규칙적인 운동 또는 적극적인 여가활동을 추구하지 않음)? ____ ____

만일 그렇지 않다면, 당신의 운동 프로그램을 기술하세요.

______________________

13. 당신은 45세 이상의 남성입니까? 또는 55세 이상의 여성입니까?

____ ____

내가 알고 있는 한, 위의 정보는 정확하며 완벽합니다.

서명________________________________________

날짜 _________________

## 정답: 문진표 작성하기

**Let me fill it out and bring it back to you!**

Name **Jennifer Karl**

Date of Birth **01/20/80**

Sex **Female** Age **31**

What is the present state of your general health?

______________________________

Physician's Name **Dr. Gopez** Phone **511-2484**

What medications are you presently taking?

**Multi vitamins**

Are you now or have you been pregnant within the past three months?

**No**

Has your physician restricted your participation in exercise?

**No**

If yes, please describe

______________________________

**Do you have now or have you ever had? Yes No**

1. A history of heart problems? _____ **No**

2. A history of lung disease? _____ **No**

3. Chest, neck, and/or jaw pains/discomforts at rest or during exertion? _____ **No**

4. Difficulty with physical exercise, such as chest pain/discomfort, dizziness or extreme shortness of breath? _____ **No**

5. Muscle, joint, or back disorder that could be aggravated by physical activity? _____ **No**

If yes, please describe ________________________________

6. A chronic illness? _____ **No**

If yes, please list ________________________________

7. High blood pressure? _____ **No**

8. Diabetes? _____ **No**

9. Cigarette-smoking habit? _____ **No**

10. High blood cholesterol? _____ **No**

11. History of heart problems in a 1st degree relative (parents, siblings, children)? _____ **No**

If yes, at what age?

Mother _____ Father _____ Brother _____ Sister _____
Son _____ Daughter _____

12. Would you describe your lifestyle as sedentary? (No regular exercise or active recreational pursuits)? _____ **No**

If no, please describe your exercise program
**I go jogging every day.**

13. Are you a male over age 45 or a female over age 55? _____ **No**

To the best of my knowledge, the above information is accurate and complete.

Signature ________________________________

Date **02/21/2011**

## 8. 전화예약: 진료예약 재 조정하기

**Receptionist:** Accurate Medical Imaging Service Center 입니다.

안녕하세요. 제가 무엇을 도와드릴까요?

**Patient:** 저는 11월 10일 오전 9시에 MRI 검사를 예약했습니다.

하지만 저는 그날 MRI 검사를 받을 수 없을 것 같습니다.

만일 가능하다면 11월 3일 오후 2시로 예약을 다시 할 수 있을까요?

**Receptionist:** 제가 그날 예약 가능한 시간이 있는지 확인해 보겠습니다.

기다려 주셔서 감사합니다. 죄송하지만 만일 예약이 취소되지 않는 한 오후 3시까지는 자리가 없습니다.

**Patient:** 음, 저는 MRI검사를 오후 3시 이후에는 언제든지 받을 수 있습니다.

**Receptionist:** 좋습니다. 3:30에 예약이 가능합니다.

이 시간으로 대신 예약 하시겠습니까?

**Patient:** 예. 아주 좋습니다. 그 시간으로 예약 하겠습니다.

**Receptionist:** 다시 확인하겠습니다.

고객님의 새 일정은 11월 3일 오후 3시 30분입니다.

**Patient:** 맞습니다. 도움 주셔서 감사합니다.

좋은 하루 되세요. 안녕히 계세요.

**Receptionist:** 선생님도요. 안녕히 계세요.

## 9. 전화예약: 응급상황

**Receptionist:** 병원입니다. 상담원 린다입니다. 무엇을 도와드릴까요?

**Patient:** 박선생님에게 진료를 보려고 예약을 하고 싶습니다.

**Receptionist**: 성함이 무엇입니까?

**Patient:** 제프리 존슨입니다.

**Receptionist:** 알겠습니다. 존슨 선생님.

어디가 아프셔서 진료를 보시려 하시나요?

**Patient:** 음, 일 주 이상을 두통으로 고생하고 있습니다.

그리고, 매일 두통이 심해지고 고열도 있습니다.

**Receptionist:** 음. 박선생님은 내일 휴진입니다.

모레까지 기다리실 수 있겠습니까?

**Patient:** 저는 오늘 꼭 진료를 보고 싶습니다.

더 이상 참을 수가 없습니다.

아마도 내가 예약없이 진료를 받을 수 있는 클리닉으로 가야만 할 것 같군요.

**Receptionist:** 잠시만요. 오늘 3시 예약이 취소 되었습니다.

내원하실 수 있습니까?

**Patient:** 지금 당장 출발하면 도착할 수 있을 것 같습니다.

**Receptionist:** 진료가 예정보다 조금 밀립니다.

그러니 세시 삼십 분경이면 박선생님에게 진료를 보실 수 있을 겁니다.

**Patient:** 정말 잘 되었네요. 그 시간으로 예약해 주셔서 감사합니다.

**Receptionist:** 천만에요. 존슨 선생님 약 한 시간 후에 뵙겠습니다

## 10. 예약관련 표현 총정리

### 진료예약없이 내원을 할 경우

1. 예약이 되어 있지는 않은데요, 너무 급합니다.

   I don't have an appointment, but it's extremely urgent.

2. 예약 없이 내원해도 됩니까?

   Could I just drop in without a scheduled appointment?

## 진료예약을 할 수 없을 경우

1. 죄송합니다만, 취소가 없는 한 11시 까지는 빈자리가 없습니다.

   I'm sorry but we don't have any openings till 11:00, unless there is a cancellation.

2. 예약일정이 내일 아침까지는 빡빡합니다. 하지만 모레에는 좀 비어 있습니다.

   Our schedule is very tight until tomorrow morning, but there are some openings in the schedule the day after tomorrow.

3. 모레까지 예약이 꽉 찼습니다.

   It's booked up till the day after tomorrow.

4. 이미 예약이 다 찼습니다.

   It's already booked up.

5. 이번 주에는 자리가 없습니다.

   We're filled up for this week.

## Chapter 1

### 의사선생님의 진료시간에 관련된 질문사항

1. Dr. Park은 12월 16일, 금요일에 진료가 없습니다.

   Dr. Park is off on Friday, December 16$^{th}$.

   Dr. Park is off duty on Friday, December 16$^{th}$.

2. Dr. Park은 휴진이십니다. Dr. Joe가 당신의 진료를 보실 것 입니다.

   Dr. Park is away. You'll be seeing Dr. Joe.

3. Dr. Joe는 12월 27일과 28일 주말에 진료를 보십니다.

   Dr. Joe is on duty over the weekends, December 27$^{th}$ and 28$^{th}$.

## 진료예약 가능한 시간/요일에 관련된 질문

1. 현재 제가 예약되어 있는 날짜보다 더 이른 날짜로 예약을 할 수 있을까요?

   Is it possible to make an appointment earlier than the one I currently have scheduled?

2. 아침 이른 시간으로 예약을 할 수 있을까요?

   Could I possibly make an appointment for early in the morning?

3. 11시 이전으로 예약 가능하겠습니까?

   Is it possible to make an appointment for earlier than 11:00?

4. 어느 시간이 좋으세요?

   What time is good for you?

5. 2시 45분 예약은 어떻습니까?

   Would 2:45 be convenient for you?
   How about 2:45?
   How does 2:45 sound?

6. 죄송하게도 오늘은 불가능하고 가장 빠른 시간은 내일 아침 9시입니다.

   I am afraid that it is booked up for today.
   The earliest opening is tomorrow morning at 9:00 a.m.

7. 어느 날이 좋으세요?

   Which day is good for you?

8. 15일 목요일로 예약 해 드릴까요?

   Can I schedule you for Thursday, the fifteenth?

9. 2월 3일 괜찮으시겠습니까?

   Is February 3rd? okay with you?

10. 가능하면 빨리 진찰을 받고 싶군요.

    I'd like to see a doctor as soon as possible.

11. 잠깐만요, 예약이 가능한지 보겠습니다.

    Just a second, please.
    Let me see if there are any openings available.

## 진료예약을 취소할 경우

1. 스케줄을 다시 잡기를 원하거나, 취소를 원하시면, 우리에게 연락을 주십시오. 전화번호는 290-6085입니다.

   If you want to reschedule or cancel your appointment, please give us a call.
   The phone number is 290-6085.

2. 만일 사정이 생겨서 예약시간에 내원하시지 못한다면, 적어도 24시간 전에는 알려주세요.

   If for any reason you are unable to make your scheduled appointment, please give a minimum of 24 hours notice.

3. 예약한 날짜에 가지 못하면 어떻게 해야 하지요?

   What if I can't make my scheduled appointment?

## Chapter 1

### 병원/클리닉 진료시간 관련 질문

1. 병원/클리닉 진료시간을 알려 주시겠습니까?

   What are the hospital hours?

   What are your clinic hours?

   What are the doctor's office hours?

## 진료예약시간 확인

1. 10시에 진료 예약을 했습니다.

   I have an appointment to see the doctor at 10:00.

2. 다음 진료예약일정은 11월 20일입니다.

   Your next appointment is scheduled on the 20th of November.

## 기타

1. 어디가 아프셔서 예약을 하십니까?

   What is the appointment regarding?

   What do you need to see the doctor about?

2. MRI검사 예약을 하려면 제 주치의 선생님의 소견서가 필요합니까?

   Do I need a referral from my primary care provider to make an appointment for an MRI exam?

3. 치과 정기검진예약을 인터넷으로 할 수 있을까요?

   Is it possible to make an appointment online for my regular dental checkup?

4. 진료일정이 약 한 시간 정도 밀려있습니다.

   We're running an hour behind schedule.

5. 예약이 취소되어 빈자리가 생기면 연락 드리겠습니다.

   We'll call you if there are any cancellations.

# Chapter 2

# Hospital/Clinic Information Desk

# 병원 안내데스크

## 1. Reading Material
독해구문

- **Hospital Information Desk, 병원 안내데스크**
- **Words, 어휘**

## Hospital Information Desk

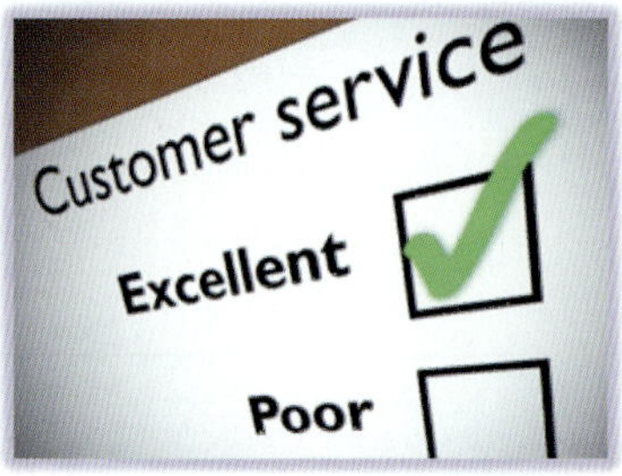


We want you to have an excellent experience at the University Hospital. If you have concern about your care, please discuss it with your physician or nurse. We also have Customer Service team members available to help you. The Customer Service team provides support to resolve your concerns. They can also arrange interpreter services, photocopying, faxing, phone access, valet car service and concierge services for out-of-town visitors. You will find Customer Service at the information desk or the Customer Service office next to Starbucks. Or, call (801) 567-2345.

## Words

* excellent: 최상의

* concern about your care: 진료에 관한 질문

* physician: 주치의

* Customer Service: 고객 서비스/고객관리

* resolve: 해결하다

* interpreter: 통역

* photocopying: 복사

* valet car service: 주차대행 서비스

* concierge service: 의전 서비스

* out-of-town visitors: 타 지역에서 오신 분들

## 2. Giving Directions to Hospitals or Clinics
병원으로 가는 길 안내

- **Directions to the University of Utah Hospital,**

  **유타대학교병원으로 가는 길**

- **Words, 어휘**

- ***Code breaker's corner: 로리와 함께 하는 미국문화 엿보기***

  - **Highway shield, 고속도로 노선번호가 삽입된 방패문양**

  - **Words, 어휘**

  - **US Map: 미국지도 및 미국 각 주의 약자 표기가 된 지도**

# Directions to the University of Utah Hospital

UNIVERSITY HOSPITAL

University Hospitals & Clinics

50 North Medical Drive

Salt Lake City, Utah 84132

Phone: (801) 581-2222

### From I-15 northbound

❶ Take the 600 South exit and go east approximately 2 miles to 700 East.

❷ Turn left and drive for five blocks until you reach 100 South.

❸ Turn right and proceed east on 100 South for one mile.

❹ When you reach the University of Utah campus, 100 South changes to North Campus Drive.

❺ Continue on North Campus Drive for one mile. University Hospital is located at 50 North Medical Drive on the right side of the street.

## Words

* Northbound: 북쪽방향, I-15=Interstate-15: 15번 고속도로

* Exit: 출구

* Turn left: 좌회전 하다

* Turn right: 우회전 하다

* Medical Drive: 병원 쪽으로 향하는 길

* Driveway: 자기집 차고로 들어가는 길

* On the right side: 오른쪽에

* **Drive** is often used for shorter stretches or streets that exist solely for access to properties: **Drive** 는 오로지 개인의 사유지에 도착하기 위한 짧은 거리(진입로) 또는 Street 을 의미합니다.

* shorter stretches: 짧은 거리(진입로)

* solely: 오로지

* access: 진입

* properties: 개인의 사유지

## *Code breaker's corner: 로리와 함께 하는 미국문화 엿보기*

### Highway shield, 고속도로 노선번호가 삽입된 방패문양

A highway shield is a sign denoting the route number of a highway, usually in the form of a symbolic shape with the route number enclosed. **Interstate 15** (I-15) is the fourth longest north–south Interstate Highway in the United States, traveling through the states of California, Nevada, Arizona, Utah, Idaho, and Montana.

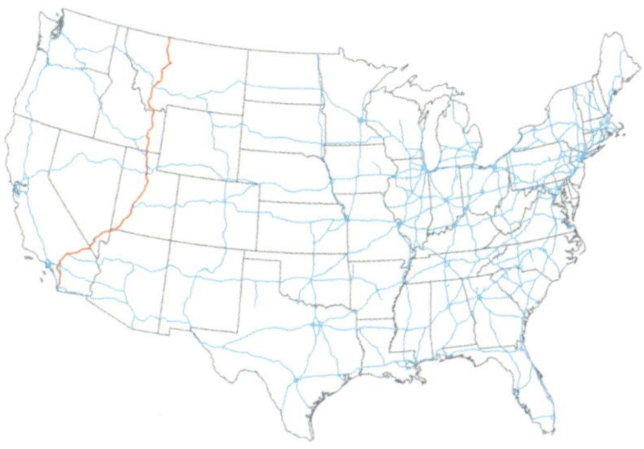

미국 I-15경로
(빨간선)

Chapter 2

## Words

* shield:  방패

* enclosed:  넣은,  포함된

* denote:  표시하다, (이름  등을)  명칭  하다.

* the fourth longest: 4 번째로  긴

* traveling through:  지나가는

## US Map

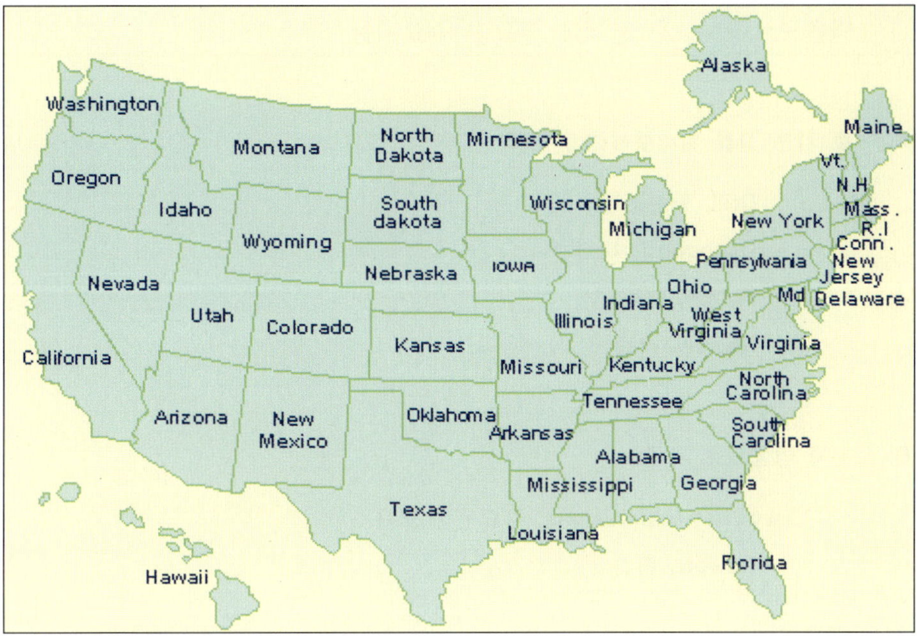


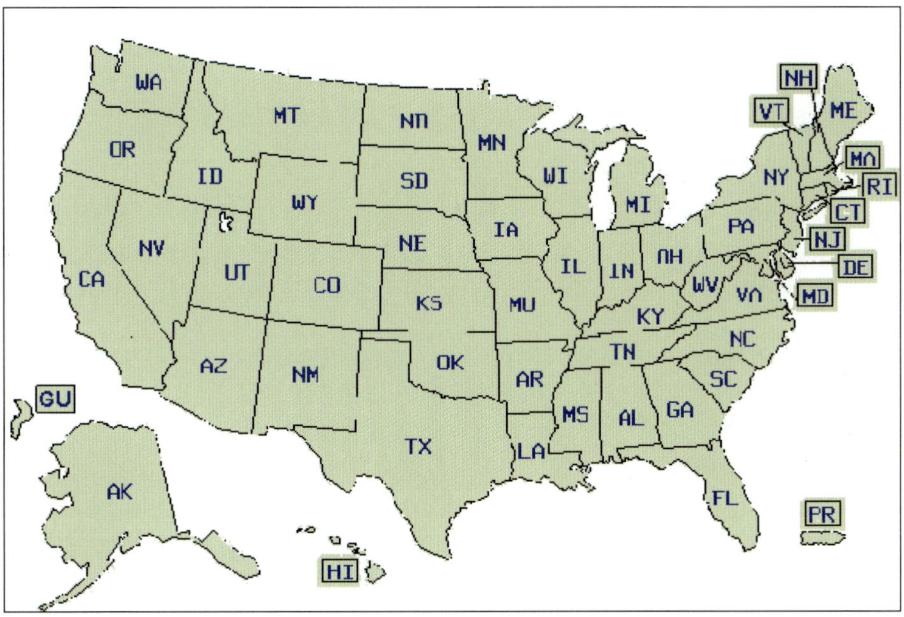


미국 주 약자 표시

## 3. Key Expressions for the Directions to the Hospital/Clinic
병원으로 가는 길 안내에 필요한 주요구문

### A. "~로 가는 길을 알려주시겠습니까?"

- Drill, 연습문제
- Dialogue 1, 대화 1
- Words, 어휘
- Review, 복습

### B. 오른쪽 방향으로 가세요

- List of Key Expressions, 주요구문 모음
  - Review, 복습

### C. 왼쪽 방향으로 가세요

- List of Key Expressions, 주요구문 모음
- Review, 복습
- Dialogue 2, 대화 2
- Words, 어휘
- Review, 복습

### D. 똑 바로 가세요.

- Dialogue 3, 대화 3
- Words, 어휘
- Review, 복습

E. 계단을 이용하세요

- Dialogue 4, 대화 4
- Words, 어휘
- Review, 복습

F. 엘리베이터를 이용하세요

- Dialogue 5, 대화 5
- Words, 어휘
- Review, 복습

G. 에스컬레이터를 이용하세요

- Dialogue 6, 대화 6
- Words, 어휘
- Review, 복습

H. 이 복도를 (쭉) 따라가세요

- Dialogue 7, 대화 7
- Words, 어휘
- Review, 복습.
- Dialogue 8, 대화 8
- Words, 어휘
- Review, 복습

I. ~을 지나가다

- Dialogue 9, 대화 9
- Words, 어휘
- Review, 복습
- Dialogue 10, 대화 10
- Words, 어휘

## Chapter 2

- **Review, 복습**

**J. ~뒤에/~앞에**

- **Dialogue 11, 대화 11**
- **Words, 어휘**
- **Review, 복습**

**K. ~의 모퉁이에**

- **Dialogue 12, 대화 12**
- **Words, 어휘**
- **Review, 복습**

**L. 대각선방향에서**

- **Definition, 의미**
- **Dialogue 13, 대화 13**
- **Dialogue 14, 대화 14**
- **Words, 어휘**
- **Review, 복습**
- **Drill, 연습문제**

---

## A. "~로 가는 길을 알려주시겠습니까?"

**Drill:** 알맞은 어휘를 아래의 Words Box에서 찾아 문장을 완성하세요.

### Words Box

* restroom
* OR (Operating Room)
* Registration Desk
* Information Desk
* pharmacy
* Discharge Department
* Medical Checkup Center
* ER (Emergency Room)
* ICU (Intensive Care Unit)

**화장실**이 어디 있는지 말해 주실래요?

Could you tell me where the ____________________ is, please?

**응급실**이 어디 있는지 말해 주실래요?

Could you tell me the way to the ______________________, please?

**접수처**가 어딘지 물어봐도 되겠어요?

May I ask you the way to the __________________________, please?

**안내데스크**가 어디에 있는지 알려주시겠습니까?

May I ask you how to get to the ________________________, please?

**퇴원계**는 어디로 가는지 말해 주시겠습니까?

Can you tell me how to get to the________________________, please?

**약국**으로 가는 길을 안내해 주시겠어요?

Could you show me the way to the ________________, please?

**중환자실**로 가는 길을 안내 해 주시겠어요?

Could you direct me to the_______________________________, please?

**건강검진센터**로 어떻게 갑니까?

How can I get to the ____________________________________, please?

이 방향이 **수술실**로 가는 길 맞습니까?

Is this the right way to the ____________________________________?

# Dialogue 1

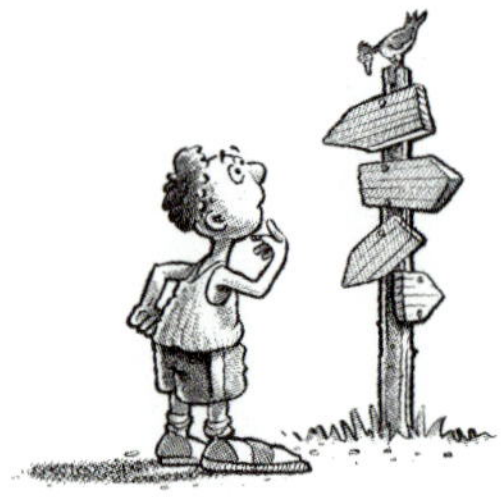

**Receptionist:** May I help you?

**Patient:** Yes. I am looking for Dr. Park's examination room. I have an appointment with him at 3:00. Could you tell me where his office is?

**Receptionist:** Sure. By the way, I am going the same way, so I will show you the way. Please come this way.

**Patient:** Wow, thanks a lot.

---

## Words

* Dr. Park's examination room: Dr. Park의 진료실

* have an appointment: 진료예약이 있다

* his office: 그의 진료실

* the same way: 같은 방향

* show you the way: 안내해 드리겠습니다

* come this way: 저를 따라오세요

**Review:** 각각의 구문을 영작하세요.
정답은 전 페이지의 Dialogue를 참고하세요.

## Dialogue 1

**Receptionist:** May I help you?

**Patient:** Yes. 저는 Dr. Park의 진료실을 찾고 있습니다.

( )

Dr. Park과 3시에 진료예약이 있습니다.

( )

Could you tell me where his office is?

**Receptionist:** Sure. 그런데 저도 같은 방향으로 갑니다.

( )

제가 안내해 드리겠습니다.

( )

저를 따라오세요

( )

**Patient:** Wow, thanks a lot.

## B. 오른쪽 방향으로 가세요

### List of Key Expressions

**Turn right: 우회전 하세요/오른쪽 방향으로 가세요**

Follow this hallway then turn right?

**Take a right/Make a right=Make a right turn: 우회전 하세요/오른쪽 방향으로 가세요**

Make a right at the corner.

Make a right turn at the traffic light.

**Turn right on 장소: 장소에서 우회전 하세요**

Go two more blocks to Avon Road and turn right on **Avon Road.**

**On the right: 오른쪽에**

It's on the right.

**On your right/on your right side: 너의 오른쪽 방향에**

CK Plastic Surgery Clinic will be on your right just past Shin-Heung Bank.

**Review:** **아래의 빈칸에 적합한 어휘를 넣어 문장을 완성하세요.**

이 복도를 따라가다 **오른쪽으로 돌아가요?**

Follow this hallway then ______________________________

**모퉁이에서** 우회전 하세요.

Make a right ______________________________

**신호등에서** 우회전 하세요.

Make a right turn ______________________________

**2블록을 더 가서** Avon Road에 도착하면 그 곳에서 우회전 하세요.

______________________to Avon Road and turn right on **Avon Road**.

**그것은 오른쪽에 있습니다.**

______________________________

CK**성형외과**는 신흥은행을 막 지나면 당신의 오른쪽 방향에 있습니다.

CK ______________ will be on your right just past Shin-Heung Bank.

## C. 왼쪽 방향으로 가세요

### List of Key Expressions

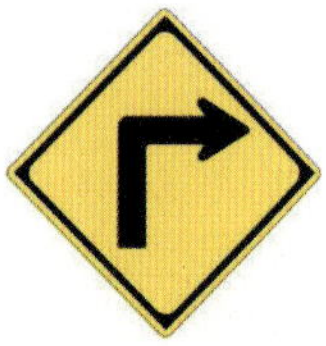

**Turn left: 좌회전 하세요/왼쪽 방향으로 가세요**

Turn left out of the elevator.

**Take a left/Make a left=Make a left turn: 좌회전 하세요/왼쪽 방향으로 가세요**

Go straight two blocks and make a left turn at the corner.

**Turn left on 장소: 장소에서 좌회전 하세요**

Turn left on **Rochester Road**.

**On the left: 왼쪽에**

The pharmacy is on the left of this hallway.

**On your left/on your left side: 너의 왼쪽 방향에**

You'll see the X-Ray room on your left side.

**Review:** 각 문장을 영작하세요.

**엘리베이터에서 내려 왼쪽 방향으로 가세요.**

____________________________________________

똑바로 두 블록 가셔서 **모퉁이에서 좌회전 하세요.**

Go straight two blocks and __________________________

Rochester Road에서 **좌회전 하세요.**

____________________________ on Rochester Road.

약국은 **이 복도의 왼쪽에** 있습니다.

The pharmacy is____________________________________

**엑스레이 검사실은 당신의 왼편에** 있습니다.

You'll see the________________________________________

# Dialogue 2

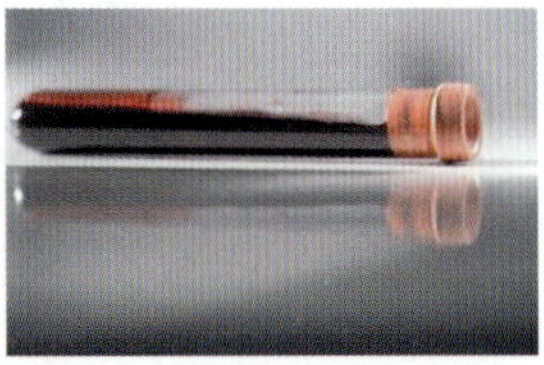

**Visitor:** Excuse me. I've heard that there's a Blood Lab nearby. Do you happen to know where it is?

**A staff member:** Sure.

Take the elevator down to the 1st floor and turn left out of the elevator.

Then, follow the hallway to the end. Blood Lab is on the right.

It's right next to the restroom. You can't miss it.

**Visitor:** Thank you so much.

**A staff member:** No problem.

---

## Words

* Blood Lab: 혈액검사실

* nearby: 근처

* Do you happen to know? : 혹시 어딘지 알고 계신가요?

* 1st floor: 1층

* You can't miss it: 바로 찾으실 거예요.

* On the south side: 남쪽에

It's on the south side of the street: 이 길의 남쪽에 위치해 있습니다.

**Review:** 각각의 구문을 영작하세요.
정답은 전 페이지의 Dialogue를 참고하세요.

## Dialogue 2

**Visitor:** Excuse me.

I've heard that there's a Blood Lab nearby.

혹시 어딘지 알고 계신가요?

( )

**A staff member:** Sure.

엘리베이터를 타고 1층에서 내려서 왼쪽으로 가세요.

( )

Then, follow the hallway to the end. Blood Lab is on the right.

화장실 바로 옆에 있습니다.

( )

You can't miss it.

**Visitor:** Thank you so much.

**A staff member:** No problem.

## D. 똑 바로 가세요

**Go straight: 똑 바로 가세요**

### Dialogue 3

**Visitor:** Excuse me.

Where is the Seoul International Medical Center?

**Local:** Well, you need to go straight two blocks on this street and make a left turn at the corner.

Then you will see a very big blue building.

That's the Seoul International Medical Center.

You can't miss it.

**Visitor:** Thanks a lot.

**Local:** Don't mention it.

---

**Words**

* visitor: 방문객

* local: 현지인.

* on this street: 이 길을 따라

* go straight: 똑 바로 가서

**Review:** 각각의 구문을 영작하세요.
**정답은 전 페이지의 Dialogue를 참고하세요.**

## Dialogue 3

**Visitor:** Excuse me.

Where is the Seoul International Medical Center?

**Local:** **이 길을 따라 똑바로 두 블록을 가셔서 모퉁이에서 좌회전 하세요.**

( )

**그러면 커다란 파란색 건물이 보입니다.**

( )

That's the Seoul International Medical Center.

**쉽게 찾으실 겁니다.**

( )

**Visitor:** Thanks a lot.

**Local:** Don't mention it.

## E. 계단을 이용하세요

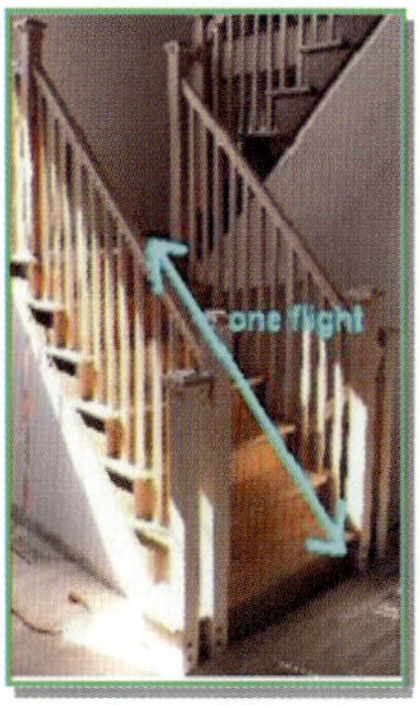


**Take the stairs.** 계단을 이용하세요.

**Go up one flight of stairs.** 계단 한 층을 올라가세요.

**Go up two flights of stairs.** 계단 두 층을 올라가세요.

**Go down one flight of stairs.** 계단 한 층을 내려가세요.

**Go down two flights of stairs.** 계단 두 층을 내려가세요.

## Dialogue 4

**Visitor:** I am looking for the Cytology Lab.

Could you tell me where it is?

**Receptionist:** Of course. It's on the third floor.

First, you need to keep following the hallway until you reach a staircase.

You are on the second floor, so you need to go up two flights of stairs to get to the third floor.

You will see the entrance door to the Cytology lab.

You can run into it.

**Visitor:** Thanks a lot. I really appreciate that.

## Words

* on the third floor: 3층에

* staircase: 계단

* hallway: 복도

* keep following the hallway: 복도를 따라 가세요

* entrance door: 입구

* You can run into it.: 쉽게 찾을 것입니다.

**Review:** 각각의 구문을 영작하세요.

정답은 전 페이지의 Dialogue를 참고하세요.

계단을 이용하세요.________________________________________

계단 한 층을 올라가세요.____________________________________

계단 두 층을 올라가세요.____________________________________

계단 한 층을 내려가세요.____________________________________

계단 두 층을 내려가세요.____________________________________

## Dialogue 4

**Visitor:** I am looking for the Cytology Lab.

Could you tell me where it is?

**Receptionist:** Of course. 삼층에 있어요.

(                                                                                                    )

First, you need to keep following the hallway until you reach a staircase.

여기가 이층이니 3층으로 가시기 위해 계단 두 층을 올라 가세요.

(                                                                                                    )

You will see the entrance door to the Cytology lab.

쉽게 찾을 것입니다.

(                                                                                                    )

**Visitor:** Thanks a lot. I really appreciate that.

## F. 엘리베이터를 이용하세요

**Take the elevator: 엘리베이터를 이용하세요**

### Dialogue 5

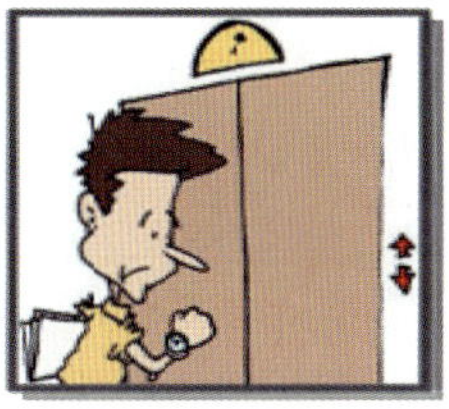

**Patient:** Do you happen to know where the Department of Otolaryngology is?

**Receptionist:** Sure. You need to take the elevator to the third floor.

Then turn left out of the elevator. It is the second door on your right.

**Patient:** Alright. So, it's on the third floor, right?

**Receptionist:** That's right. It's on the third floor.

**Patient:** I got it. Thank you, ma'am.

**Receptionist:** You're welcome.

---

### Words

* Otolaryngology=Otorhinolaryngology 이비인후과

* take the elevator to the third floor:
  엘리베이터를 타고 3층으로 올라가세요

* second door on your right. : 당신의 오른쪽에서 두 번째 방

* I got it: 알겠습니다.

**Review:** 각각의 구문을 영작하세요.
정답은 전 페이지의 Dialogue를 참고하세요.

## Dialogue 5

**Patient:** 이비인후과가 어디에 있는지 혹시 알고 계십니까?

( )

**Receptionist:** Sure. 엘리베이터를 타고 3층으로 올라가세요.

( )

Then turn left out of the elevator.

당신의 오른쪽에서 두 번째 방입니다.

( )

**Patient:** Alright. So, it's on the third floor, right?

**Receptionist:** That's right. It's on the third floor.

**Patient:** I got it. Thank you, ma'am.

**Receptionist:** You're welcome.

## G. 에스컬레이터를 이용하세요

**Take the escalator up two flights:** 에스컬레이터를 타고 두 층을 올라가세요.

**Take the escalator down one level:** 에스컬레이터를 타고 한 층 내려가세요.

## Dialogue 6

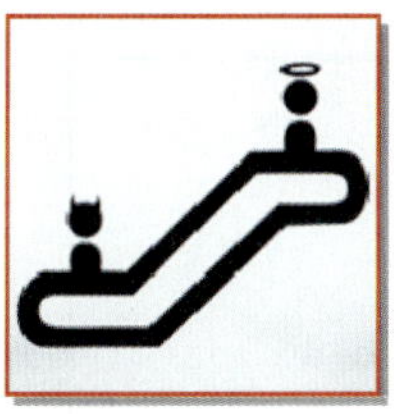

**Receptionist:** Could I help you?

**Visitor:** Yes. Could you tell me where I can find Starbucks?

**Receptionist:** Sure. There's one on the lobby.

Take the escalator down one level and turn right.

Then, proceed to the Information Desk.

The Starbucks is right next to the Information Desk.

**Visitor:** Thanks a lot!

**Receptionist:** You are more than welcome.

### Words

* proceed to: ~로 가세요.

* Information Desk: 안내데스크

* right next to ~: ~ 바로 옆에

* You are more than welcome/You are welcome: 천만에요.

Chapter 2

**Review:** 각각의 구문을 영작하세요.
정답은 전 페이지의 Dialogue를 참고하세요.

에스컬레이터를 타고 두 층을 올라가세요.______________________

______________________________________________

에스컬레이터를 타고 한 층 내려가세요.______________________

______________________________________________

## Dialogue 6

**Receptionist:** Could I help you?

**Visitor:** Yes. Could you tell me where I can find Starbucks?

**Receptionist:** Sure. 로비에 있습니다.

( )

에스컬레이터를 타고 한층 내려가셔서 오른쪽으로 가세요.

( )

그런 후, 안내데스크로 가세요.

( )

The Starbucks is right next to the Information Desk.

**Visitor:** Thanks a lot!

**Receptionist:** You are more than welcome.

## H. 이 복도를 따라가세요

**Follow this hallway:** 이 복도를 따라가세요

**Go (straight) down the hallway:** 이 복도를 (쭉) 따라가세요

### Dialogue 7

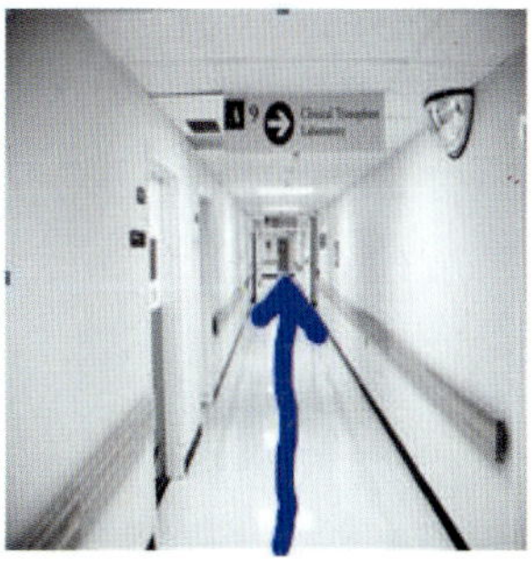

**Visitor:** I am looking for the Pediatric Cardiology Center. Do you happen to know where it is?

**A staff member:** Yes, I do. Follow this hallway. When you reach the end of the hallway, go to your left. Then the Pediatric Cardiology Center will be the second door on the left.

**Visitor:** I am sorry, but I couldn't follow you. Could you repeat that please?

**A staff member:** Sure. Follow this hallway to the end. Then go to your left.

**Visitor:** Follow this hallway to the end and make a left turn?

**A staff member:** That's right. Then the Pediatric Cardiology Center will be the second door on the left.

**Visitor:** I see. I really appreciate that.

**A staff member:** Don't mention it.

Chapter 2

## Words

* Pediatric Cardiology Center: 소아심장센터

* the end of the hallway: 복도 끝

* I couldn’t follow you: 이해가 안됐어요.

**Review:** 각각의 구문을 영작하세요.
정답은 전 페이지의 Dialogue를 참고하세요.

### Dialogue 7

**Visitor:** 저는 소아심장센터를 찾고 있습니다.

( )

Do you happen to know where it is?

**A staff member:** Yes, I do. Follow this hallway.

복도 끝에 도달하면 왼쪽으로 가세요.

( )

Then the Pediatric Cardiology Center will be the second door on the left.

**Visitor:** 미안하지만, 이해가 안됐어요.

( )

Could you repeat that please?

**A staff member:** Sure. 이 복도 끝까지 따라가세요.

( )

그리고 왼쪽으로 가세요. ( )

**Visitor:** 이 복도를 따라가다가 왼쪽으로 가요?

( )

**A staff member:** That's right. Then the Pediatric Cardiology Center will be the second door on the left.

**Visitor:** I see. I really appreciate that.

**A staff member:** Don't mention it.

# Dialogue 8

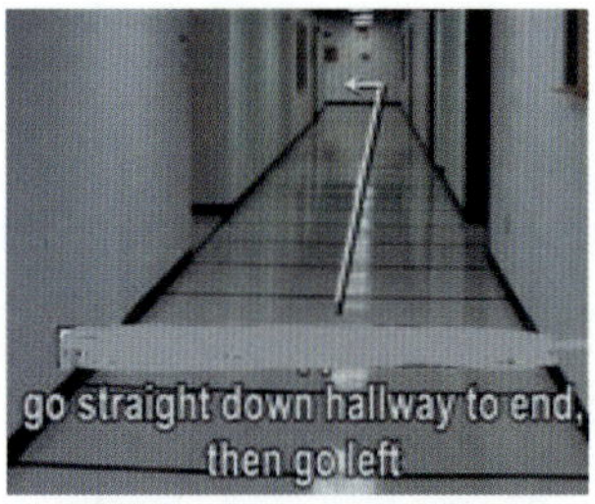


**Visitor:** Excuse me.

I am looking for an elevator.

Is there an elevator near here?

**John Doe:** Yes. There is one down there.

You need to go straight down the hallway to the end and go left. Then, you will see the visitor's elevator.

**Visitor:** I need to go to the end of the hallway, right?

**John Doe:** That's right, sir.

**Visitor:** Thanks a lot.

**John Doe:** No problem.

## Words

* There is: ~이 있다.

* John Doe: 홍길동

* the visitor's elevator: 방문객 전용 엘리베이터

* go straight down the hallway: 복도 끝까지 따라 가다

**Review:** 각각의 구문을 영작하세요.
정답은 전 페이지의 Dialogue를 참고하세요.

## Dialogue 8

**Visitor:** Excuse me.

I am looking for an elevator.

이 근처에 엘리베이터가 있나요?

( )

**John Doe:** Yes. 저쪽 끝에 있어요.

( )

복도 끝까지 따라 가셔서 왼쪽으로 가세요.

( )

Then, you will see the visitor's elevator.

**Visitor:** I need to go to the end of the hallway, right?

**John Doe:** That's right, sir.

**Visitor:** Thanks a lot.

**John Doe:** No problem.

## I. ~을 지나가다

**Go past~/Pass: ~을 지나가다**

### Dialogue 9

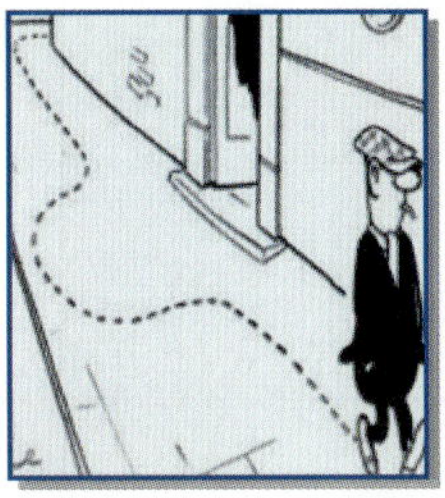

**Visitor:** Excuse me. How do I get to the Medical Plaza?

**Local:** Keep going down this street until you reach the post office. Then turn left at the post office.

**Visitor:** Okay.

**Local:** After turning left, go past the library and it's right next to the library.

**Visitor:** Is it far from here?

**Local:** Not really.

**Visitor:** I see. Thank you so much.

**Local:** You are welcome.

---

**Words**

* post office: 우체국

* far: 먼 (거리상)

* right next to: 바로 옆

**Review:** 각각의 구문을 영작하세요.
정답은 전 페이지의 Dialogue를 참고하세요.

## Dialogue 9

**Visitor:** Excuse me. How do I get to the Medical Plaza?

**Local:** 우체국에 도착할 때까지 이 길을 따라 계속 가세요.

( )

Then turn left at the post office.

**Visitor:** Okay.

**Local:** 좌회전한 후에, 도서관을 지나세요. 그러면 도서관 바로 옆 건물이에요.

( )

**Visitor:** 여기에서 먼가요?

( )

**Local:** Not really.

**Visitor:** I see. Thank you so much.

**Local:** You are welcome.

# Dialogue 10

**Patient:** Would you please tell me where the Radiology Department is?

**Receptionist:** Sure.

Keep walking until you pass the ER (Emergency Room).

Then, you will see the Radiology Department right next to the ER (Emergency Room).

**Patient:** Oh, I see. Thanks a lot.

**Receptionist:** You are welcome.

## Words

* Radiology Department: 영상의학과

* until: ~ 때까지

* ER (Emergency Room): 응급실

**Review:** 각각의 구문을 영작하세요.
**정답은 전 페이지의 Dialogue를 참고하세요.**

## Dialogue 10

**Patient:** 영상의학과가 어디에 있는지 말씀해 주시겠습니까?

( )

**Receptionist:** Sure. 응급실을 지날 때까지 계속 가세요.

( )

그러면 영상의학과가 응급실 바로 옆에 있는 것을 보시게 될 것입니다.

( )

**Patient:** Oh, I see. Thanks a lot.

**Receptionist:** You are welcome.

## J. ~뒤에/~앞에

**Behind:** ~뒤에

**In front of:** ~앞에

### Dialogue 11

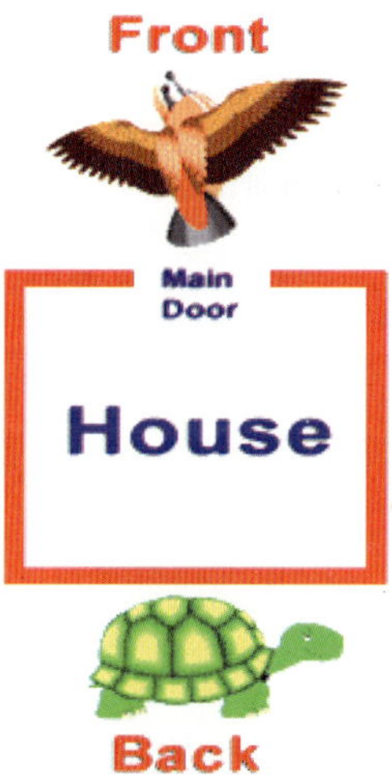


**Patient:** Excuse me.

Do you know where the consultation room is?

**Nurse:** Of course. It is in front of the doctor's examination room.

**Patient:** Thanks a lot. By the way, could you tell me where the nearest bank is, too?

**Nurse:** Sure. It is located behind the main hospital building.

---

### Words

* consultation room: 진료상담실

* doctor's examination room: 진료실

* the nearest: 가장 가까운

* main hospital building: 본관

**Review:** 각각의 구문을 영작하세요.
정답은 전 페이지의 Dialogue를 참고하세요.

## Dialogue 11

**Patient:** Excuse me.

진료상담실이 어디에 있는지 아십니까?

( )

**Nurse:** Of course. 진료실 앞에 있습니다.

( )

**Patient:** Thanks a lot.

By the way, could you tell me where the nearest bank is, too?

**Nurse:** Sure. 본관 뒤에 있습니다.

( )

## K. ~의 모퉁이에

**At the corner/On the corner: ~의 모퉁이에**

### Dialogue 12

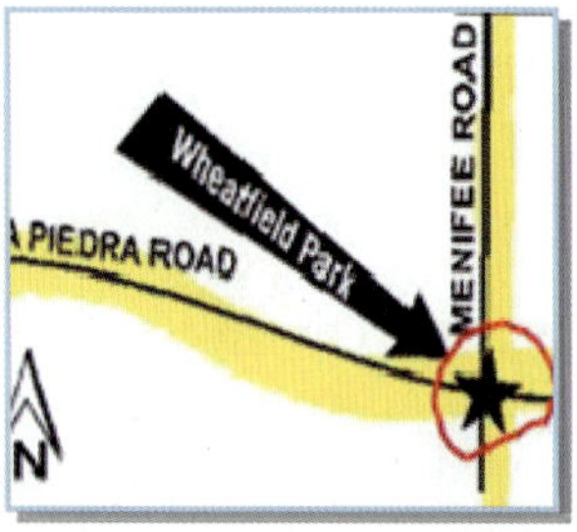


**Visitor:** Can you tell me how to get to the Kyung Hee University International Medical Service (**KUIMS**)?

**Jane Doe:** Sure.

**Visitor:** Is it far from here?

**Jane Doe:** Not really. Go straight down this street for two blocks. Then turn left. You will see the Kyung Hee University International Medical Service (**KUIMS**) at the corner.

**Visitor:** Thanks a lot.

**Jane Doe:** You are more than welcome.

### Words

* how to get to: ~로 가는 방법

* Just around the corner: 가까이에, 이 근처에

There's a good restaurant just around the corner.

좋은 레스토랑이 이 근처에 있어요.

Christmas is just around the corner.

크리스마스가 얼마 안 남았네요.

**Review:** 각각의 구문을 영작하세요.

정답은 전 페이지의 Dialogue를 참고하세요.

## Dialogue 12

**Visitor:** Can you tell me how to get to the Kyung Hee International Medical Service (**KUIMS**)?

**Jane Doe:** Sure.

**Visitor:** 여기에서 먼가요?

( )

**Jane Doe:** Not really. 이 길을 따라 두 블록을 더 가세요.

( )

Then turn left. 강동경희대병원 국제 클리닉센터는 길 모퉁이에 있을 것입니다.

( )

**Visitor:** Thanks a lot.

**Jane Doe:** You are more than welcome.

## L. ~대각선방향에서

**Caddy corner from ~: ~대각선 방향에서**

**Definition:** It is diagonally opposite from the point where you are now, as if standing on one corner in a square.

"There is a house that sits caddy corner from the 4-H center."

### Dialogue 13

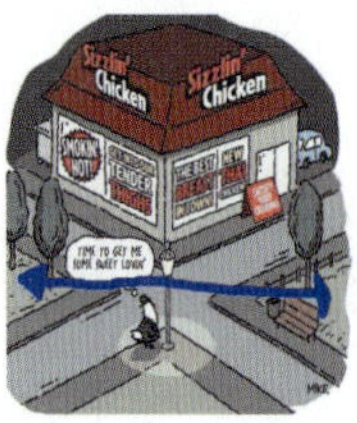


**Visitor:** Where is the post office?

**John Doe:** It's caddy corner from this building.

### Dialogue 14

**Jane Doe:** Could you tell me where I can find a children's bookstore around here?

**Local:** Sure. The children's bookstore sits caddy corner from the library on Adams Avenue.

---

**Words**

* diagonally: 대각선으로
* opposite: ~과 반대
* Jane Doe: 홍길순
* square: 사각형

**Review:** 각각의 구문을 영작하세요.
정답은 전 페이지의 Dialogue를 참고하세요.

## Dialogue 13

**Visitor:** Where is the post office?

**John Doe:** 이 건물에서 대각선 방향에 있습니다.

( )

## Dialogue 14

**Jane Doe:** Could you tell me where I can find a children's bookstore around here?

**Local:** Sure. 어린이책 서점은 아담스 에비뉴에 있는 도서관의 대각선 방향에 위치해 있습니다.

( )

**Drill:** 아래의 글을 읽고 Bank of America의 위치를 그리세요.

Rehab center is at the corner of Churchville Rd. and Main St.

Bank of America is caddy corner from Rehab center.

* Road의 약자: Rd.

* Street의 약자: St.

## 4. Drill
연습문제

- **Drill: This is your last stop for ~, 에 관한 최고의 상점입니다.**

- **Words, 어휘**

**Drill:** 아래에 설명된 가게를 지도에서 찾아 동그라미를 치세요.

**This is your last stop for** replacing watch batteries, watch and clock repair, restoration and jewelry repair in Portland, Oregon.

You can find us **on the corner of** Laurel Wood & Beaverton-Hillsdale and **caddy corner from** US bank.

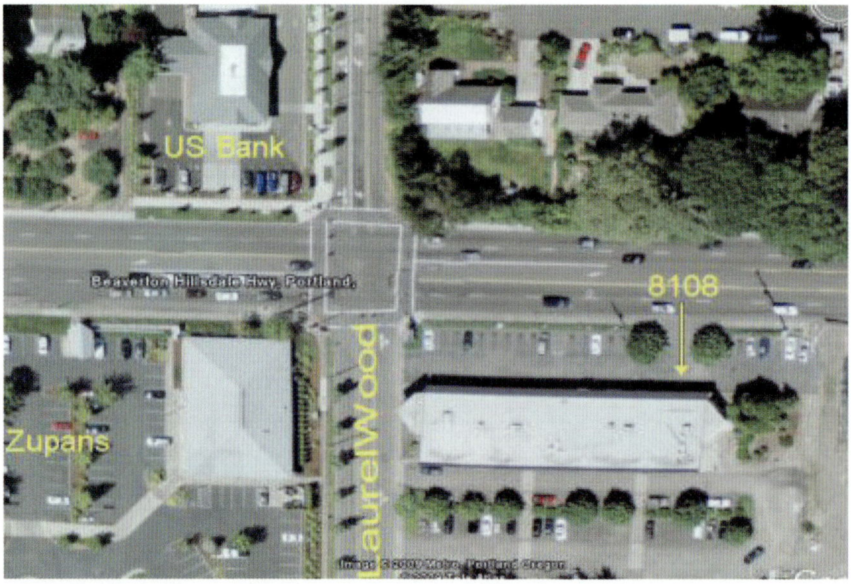


아래의 문장을 해석하세요.

Make Us Your First And Last Stop For All of Your Medical Supply Needs.

## Words

* Your last stop: 모든 것을 할 수 있는 곳.

* replacing watch batteries: 시계건전지 교체

* watch: 손목시계

* repair: 수리

* restoration: 복원

* jewelry: 보석

* your first and last stop: 모든 것을 판매하며 최고의 서비스를 제공하는 곳

## 5. Key Expressions
주요구문

- **Drill, 연습문제**

**Drill: 아래의 질문을 영작하세요.**

Q1: 그건 약국 **앞에** 있어요.

A1: It's______________________the pharmacy.

Q2: University Street에 **하나 있어요.**

A2: ____________________on the University Street

Q3: 저는 **피부과를** 찾고 잇습니다.

A3: I'm looking for_____________________.

Q4: **재활센터는 길 건너편에** 있어요.

A4: _________________________is______________________.

* across from ~: ~(건물 또는 대상) 건너편에
* across the street: 길 건너편에 (건물 또는 대상의 건너편이 아닌, 길 건너편일 경우 from을 사용하지 않음)

Q5: LK 한의원으로 가는 **지름길**을 알려주세요.

A5: Could you tell me ___________________to get to LK Korean Medicine Clinic?

* shortcut/the shortest route: 지름길

## Chapter 2

Q6: **외래환자 클리닉 입구**는 어디입니까?

A6: Where is__________________________________?

Q7: **입원 환자 병동**을 가르쳐 주시겠어요?

A7: Could you tell me where ____________________is?

Q8: **외과 병동**의 몇 호실 입니까?

A8: Which room is it in______________________________?

Q9: **복도 중간에** 있어요.

A9: It's________________________________.

Q10: **세 번째 방까지 가서 오른쪽**으로 가세요.

A10: You need to walk down to_________________________________.

Q 11: **3호선 지하철** 타는 곳을 알려주시겠습니까?

A11: Could you tell me where I can take_____________________?

Q 12: 잠실 역에서 내려서 **10번 출구로 가세요**.

A 12: You need to get off at the Jamsil Station and then _______________

__________________________________

## 6. Business, Hospital and Clinic Hours
병원시설 업무시간과 병원진료시간

A. Eateries, 식당가

- Cafeteria, 구내식당
  - Dialogue 1, 대화 1
  - Words, 어휘
  - Review, 복습
- Starbucks, 스타벅스
  - Dialogue 2, 대화 2
  - Words, 어휘
  - Review, 복습

B. Hospital Hours/Clinic hours, 진료시간

- Beta Clinic Hours
  - Dialogue 3, 대화 3
  - Words, 어휘
  - Review, 복습
- Drill, 연습문제
  - Words, 어휘

C. Directory, 병원층별 안내

- Words, 어휘
- Dialogue 4, 대화 4
- Words, 어휘
- Review, 복습

Chapter 2

## A. Eateries

### Cafeteria

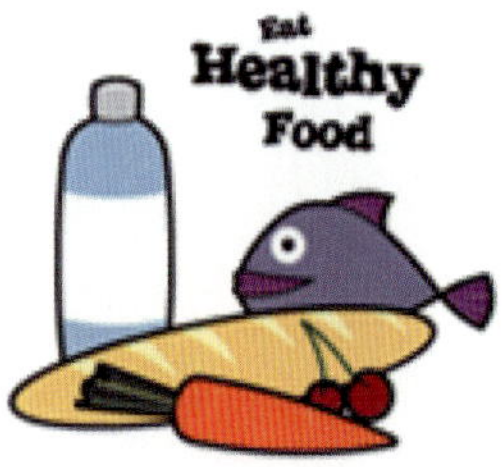


**CAFETERIA**

Level A. Breakfast, Lunch and Dinner.

Hours: Mon. – Fri. 6:30 a.m. – 10 p.m.,

Sat. – Sun. and holidays 8 a.m. – 8 p.m.

### Dialogue 1

**Receptionist:** Cafeteria. How may I help you today?

**Customer:** What are your business hours?

**Receptionist:** Okay. We are open Monday through Friday, 6:30 a.m. to 10 p.m.

On Saturdays, Sundays and holidays, we are open from 8 a.m. to 8 p.m.

Is there anything else that I can help you with?

**Customer:** Not really. Thank you for your help.

## Words

* Hours: (구내식당) 영업시간

* Mon. – Fri.: 월요일부터 금요일까지

* 6:30 a.m. – 10 p.m.: 오전 6:30부터 오후 10:00까지

* holidays: 공휴일

* business hours: 영업시간

Chapter 2

**Review:** 각각의 구문을 영작하세요.
정답은 전 페이지의 Dialogue를 참고하세요.

## Dialogue 1

**Receptionist:** Cafeteria. How may I help you today?

**Customer:** 영업시간이 어떻게 되나요?
( )

**Receptionist:** Okay. 월요일부터 금요일까지는 오전 6:30부터 오후 10:00까지 문을 엽니다.
( )

토요일, 일요일, 그리고 공휴일에는 오전 8:00에서 오후 8:00까지 문을 엽니다.
( )

Is there anything else that I can help you with?

**Customer:** Not really. Thank you for your help.

## Starbucks

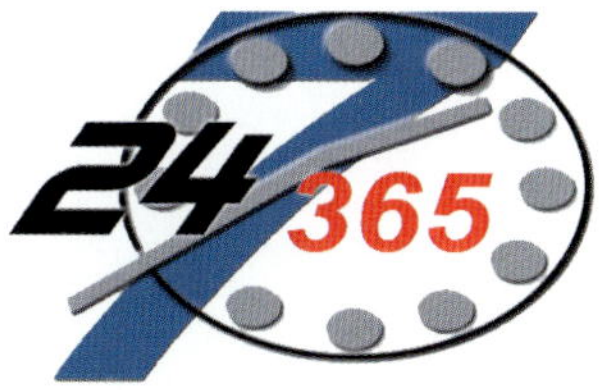


Located on **Level 1** near the lobby

Open 24 hours a day, 7 days a week

## Dialogue 2

**Receptionist:** Starbucks. How may I help you?

**Visitor:** Yes. I'd like to know your business hours, please.

**Receptionist:** Sure. We are open 24 hours a day, 7 days a week. We are always here for you.

**Visitor:** Wow. It's 24/7 (twenty four-seven), right?

**Receptionist:** That's right. Do you have other questions to ask?

**Visitor:** Yes. What is your location, please?

**Receptionist:** We are located on Level 1 near the lobby.

**Visitor:** I see. I'll stop by in a minute.

**Receptionist:** Alright, see you soon.

## Chapter 2

---

### Words

* 24/7/365 하루 24시간 주 7일, 연중무휴 운영한다는 뜻.

* 24/7은 twenty four-seven 으로 읽습니다.

* around the clock: 24시간 내내

* stop by: 들르다

* in a minute: 곧

**Review:** 각각의 구문을 영작하세요.
정답은 전 페이지의 Dialogue를 참고하세요.

## Dialogue 2

**Receptionist:** Starbucks. How may I help you?

**Visitor:** Yes. I'd like to know your business hours, please.

**Receptionist:** Sure. 우리는 하루 24시간 주 7일 열고 있습니다.

( )

We are always here for you.

**Visitor:** Wow. 연중 무휴이군요. 그렇지요?

( )

**Receptionist:** That's right. Do you have other questions to ask?

**Visitor:** Yes. What is your location, please?

**Receptionist:** 우리는 Level 1 의 로비 근처에 위치해 있습니다.

( )

**Visitor:** I see. 곧 들르겠습니다.

( )

**Receptionist:** Alright, see you soon.

## B. Hospital Hours/Clinic hours

### Beta Clinic Hours

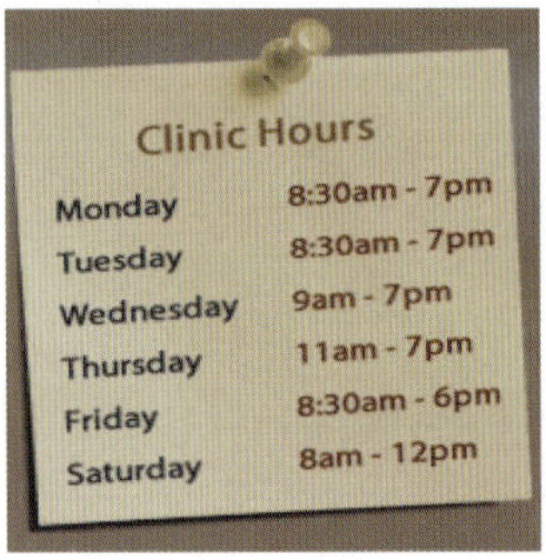


The clinic operates on an appointment system, or on a drop-in basis.

For an appointment, please call at this number 476-8976.

### Dialogue 3

**Patient:** What are your clinic hours?

**Receptionist:** Our clinic hours are 8:00 a.m. to 4:00 p.m., Monday through Friday. Do you have an appointment with us?

**Patient:** No, I don't. But I'd like to make an appointment to see a doctor.

**Receptionist:** Then, you need to call at this number to make an appointment. The number is 476-8976.

**Patient:** Thank you for your help. I really appreciate that.

**Receptionist:** You are welcome.

## Words

* Clinic Hours: 클리닉 진료시간

* operates on: 진료를 받을 수 있습니다.

* appointment system: 예약제

* drop-in basis: 예약 없이

* A drop-in basis, meaning you do not have to tell us when you come or leave:
예약 없이도 내원가능, 언제 오거나 가는 시간을 우리에게 말할 필요가 없는 뜻.

All our classes are on a drop–in basis: 우리의 모든 수업은 예약 없이 들을 수 있습니다.

**Review:** 각각의 구문을 영작하세요.
정답은 전 페이지의 Dialogue를 참고하세요.

## Dialogue 3

**Patient:** 진료시간이 어떻게 되지요?

( )

**Receptionist:** 우리의 진료시간은 월요일부터 금요일, 오전 8시부터 오후 4시입니다.

( )

저희 클리닉과 예약을 하셨나요?

( )

**Patient:** No, I don't. 하지만 진료를 보기 위해 예약을 하고 싶습니다.
( )
**Receptionist:** Then, you need to call at this number to make an appointment. The number is 476-8976.

**Patient:** Thank you for your help. I really appreciate that.

**Receptionist:** You are welcome.

**Drill:** 아래의 진료시간을 보고 질문 1-5에 답하세요.

**Flu Clinics at the Utah County Health Department (UCHD)*:**
**(The Utah County Health and Justice Building, 151 South University Avenue, Provo)**

| Monday | Tuesday | Wednesday | Thursday | Friday |
|---|---|---|---|---|
| 8am - 4:30pm | 8am - 4:30pm | 8am - 7:00pm | 9am - 4:30pm | 8am - 4:30pm |

**Other-site Flu Clinics Options*:**
**(All Other-site Clinics are by appointment unless otherwise noted. Please call 851-7025.)**

| | |
|---|---|
| American Fork Hospital<br>120 N 1220 E #10, American Fork | Mondays, 3-7pm flu walk-ins welcome |
| Orem Community Hospital<br>331 N 400 W, Orem | 1st and 3rd Thursdays, 2:30pm - 4:30pm* |
| Payson City Center<br>439 W Utah Ave, Payson | Tuesdays, 5pm - 7pm* |
| Saratoga Springs Instanta Care<br>250 E State Road 73, Saratoga Springs | 2nd and 4th Thursdays, 2:30pm - 4:30pm* |

* excludes holidays
⌘ by appointment, please call 851-7025

## Words

* Flu clinic: 독감예방주사를 맞을 수 있는 클리닉

* Other-site Flu Clinics Options: 독감예방주사를 맞을 수 있는 다른 지역의 클리닉들

* unless otherwise noted: 다른 공지 사항이 없는 한

* All other-site Clinics are by appointment unless otherwise noted: 다른 공지사항이 없는 한 타 지역의 모든 클리닉들은 예약을 해야 합니다.

* exclude holidays: 공휴일을 제외한

* by appointment, please call 851-7025: 예약을 하려면 851-7025로 전화하세요.

## Chapter 2

1. 진료예약 없이 독감예방주사를 맞을 수 있는 클리닉의 장소를 적으세요.

2. 독감예방주사를 맞기 위해 사전 진료예약을 요구하는 클리닉을 모두 적으세요.

3. 사전예약이 요구되고 저녁시간에 독감주사를 맞을 수 있는 클리닉은 무슨 요일에 내원 가능한가요?

4. 토요일에 독감예방주사를 맞을 수 있는 클리닉의 위치를 모두 적으세요.

5. 독감예방주사를 맞기 위한 진료예약을 할 때 사용하는 클리닉 전화번호를 적으세요.

## C. Directory

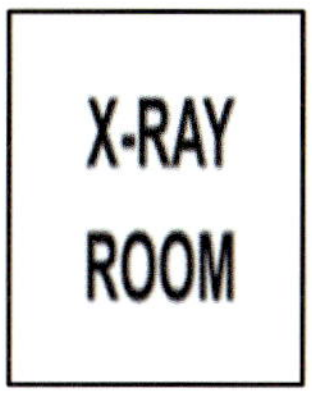


**Patient:** Could you tell me how to get to the X-ray room?

**Receptionist:** Yes. First, you need to follow this hallway to the end. Then the X-ray room is right next to the ER (Emergency Room).

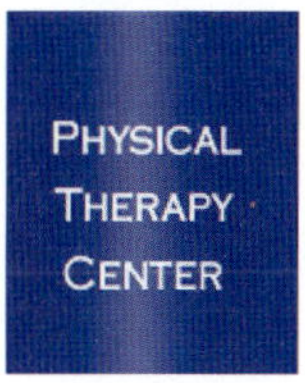


**Patient:** Excuse me. Can you tell me where the physical therapy center is?

**Receptionist:** Sure. From the disabled entrance, go down two flights of stairs. Then it will be the second door on the left. You can't miss it.

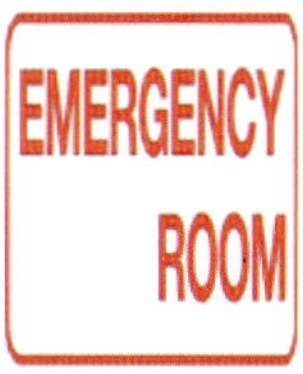


**Patient:** Can you direct me to the ER (Emergency Room)?

**Receptionist:** Alright. The ER (Emergency Room) is located on the first floor. It's right next to the CT scan room.

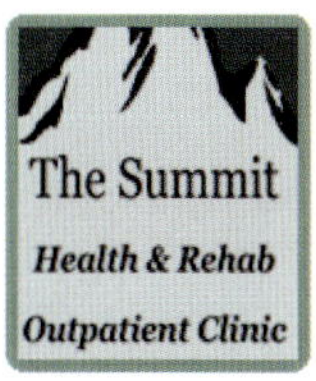


**Patient:** How do I get to the Outpatient Clinic?

**Receptionist:** It's on the second floor. Take the elevator to the second floor. Then, turn left out of the elevator and follow the yellow arrow on the floor.

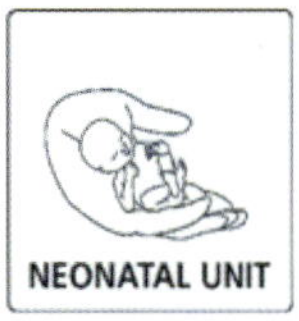


**Patient:** Where is the Neonatal Care Unit?

**Receptionist:** It's on the 3rd floor.
It's across from the Delivery Room.

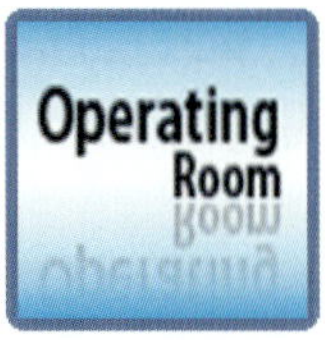


**Patient:** Is there an Operating Room near here?

**Receptionist:** Yes. There's one on the third floor.
It's right across from the ICU (Intensive Care Unit).

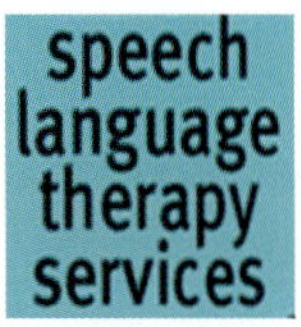


**Patient:** I wonder if you could help me.
I'm looking for the Speech Therapy Room.

**Receptionist:** It's right next to the Physical Therapy Room.

---

## Words

* Directory: 안내도(층별 안내도)

* X-ray room/X-ray lab: 엑스레이 검사실

* right next to: ~ 바로 옆에

* Outpatient Clinic: 외래진료소

* Delivery Room: 분만실

# Dialogue 4

**Receptionist:** How can I help you?

**Visitor:** I am looking for Huntsman Cancer Institute.

**Receptionist:** I see. You need to take the visitor's elevator to the 3rd floor. Then turn right out of the elevator. Keep going until you pass Clinical Neurosciences Center. And then, you'll see Huntsman Cancer Institute on your left side. Are you with me so far?

**Visitor:** I am afraid not. Would you say that again, please?

**Receptionist:** Sure. First, take the visitor's elevator to the 3rd floor.

**Visitor:** Um. Where is the visitor's elevator?

**Receptionist:** It's right next to the Starbucks in the lobby.

**Visitor:** I need to take the visitor's elevator right next to the Starbucks in the lobby and then get off on the 3rd floor, right?

**Receptionist:** That's right. Next, you need to follow the hallway until you pass Clinical Neurosciences Center.

Then, Huntsman Cancer Institute will be on your left side.

You will run into it.

**Visitor:** Okay. I follow down the hallway to reach the Clinical Neurosciences Center. Then, I will see the Huntsman Cancer Institute on my left side, right?

**Receptionist:** You got it right.

**Visitor:** Thank you so much. I really appreciate it.

Chapter 2

## Words

* visitor's elevator: 방문객 전용 엘리베이터

* Are you with me so far? 이해가 되십니까?

* I am afraid not: 죄송합니다만, 이해가 잘 안돼요.

* get off on the 3rd floor: 3층에서 내리다.

* reach: ~에 도달하다.

**Review:** 각각의 구문을 영작하세요.
**정답은 전 페이지의 Dialogue를 참고하세요.**

## Dialogue 4

**Receptionist:** How can I help you?

**Visitor:** I am looking for Huntsman Cancer Institute.

**Receptionist:** I see. **방문객 전용 엘리베이터를 타고 3층으로 가세요.**
( )

Then turn right out of the elevator. Keep going until you pass Clinical Neurosciences Center.

And then, you'll see Huntsman Cancer Institute on your left side.

**이해가 되십니까?**
( )

**Visitor:** **죄송합니다만, 이해가 잘 안돼요.**
( )

Would you say that again, please?

**Receptionist:** Sure. First, take the visitor's elevator to the 3rd floor.

**Visitor:** Um. Where is the visitor's elevator?

**Receptionist:** It's right next to the Starbucks near the lobby.

**Visitor: 로비에 있는 스타벅스 바로 옆에 있는 방문객 전용 엘리베이터를 타고 3층에서 내리는 거죠. 그렇지요?**

( )

**Receptionist:** That's right. Next, you need to follow the hallway until you pass Clinical Neurosciences Center.

Then, Huntsman Cancer Institute will be on your left side.

**금방 찾으실 것입니다.**

( )

**Visitor:** Okay. I follow down the hallway to reach the Clinical Neurosciences Center. Then, I will see the Huntsman Cancer Institute on my left side, right?

**Receptionist: 맞아요.**

( )

**Visitor:** Thank you so much. I really appreciate it.

# 7. Parking Services
주차안내

- **Self Parking, 자가주차**
- **Words, 어휘**
- **Dialogue 1, 대화 1**
- **Words, 어휘**
- **Review, 복습**
- **Valet Parking, 주차대행 서비스**
- **Words, 어휘**
- **Dialogue 2, 대화 2**
- **Words, 어휘**
- **Review, 복습**
- **Drill, 연습문제**
- **Words, 어휘**

Chapter 2

## Self Parking

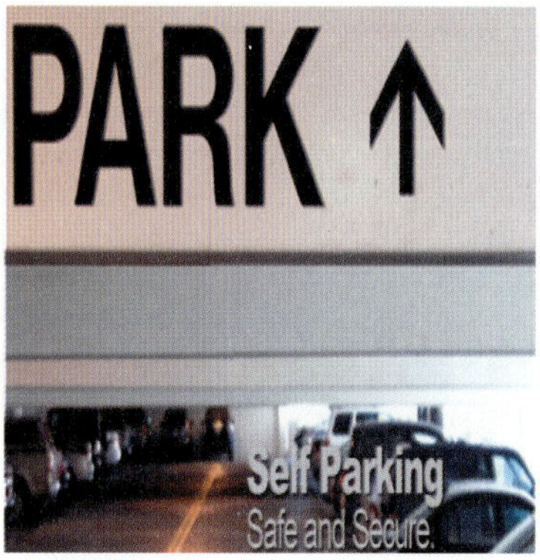


If you prefer to park your vehicle on your own, free self parking is available in our patient/visitor parking terrace located on the right side of the hospital driveway just as you enter. Please remember to make note of where you parked your vehicle and what hospital entrance you used.

### Words

* Self Parking: 자가주차

* vehicle: 자동차

* parking terrace: 주차장

* hospital driveway: 병원으로 향하는 길/진입로

* hospital entrance: 병원의 출입문

# Dialogue 1

**Visitor:** Excuse me. Is there a parking lot near here?

**Local:** Yes. There is one near the hospital driveway.

**Visitor:** Is it difficult to find it? Because I am new here.

**Local:** Not at all. There are signs for the parking lot.

Actually, they are right in front of you.

You can follow the signs. It's pretty easy.

**Visitor:** By the way, is it free of charge?

**Local:** Yes, it is.

**Visitor:** I see. Thanks a lot.

---

## Words

* parking lot: 주차장

* I am new here: 제가 이곳을 처음 방문해서요.

* signs for the parking lot: 주차장으로 가는 표식

* right in front of you: 바로 앞에

* follow the signs: 표식을 따라가세요

* free of charge: 무료

Chapter 2

**Review:** 각각의 구문을 영작하세요.
정답은 전 페이지의 Dialogue를 참고하세요.

### Dialogue 1

**Visitor:** Excuse me. 이 근처에 주차장이 있나요?
( )

**Local:** Yes. There is one near the hospital driveway.

**Visitor:** Is it difficult to find it? 제가 이곳을 처음 방문해서요.
( )

**Local:** Not at all. There are signs for the parking lot.

Actually, they are right in front of you.

표식을 따라가세요.

( )

It's pretty easy.

**Visitor:** 그런데, 주차비는 무료입니까?
( )

**Local:** Yes, it is.

**Visitor:** I see. Thanks a lot.

## Valet Parking

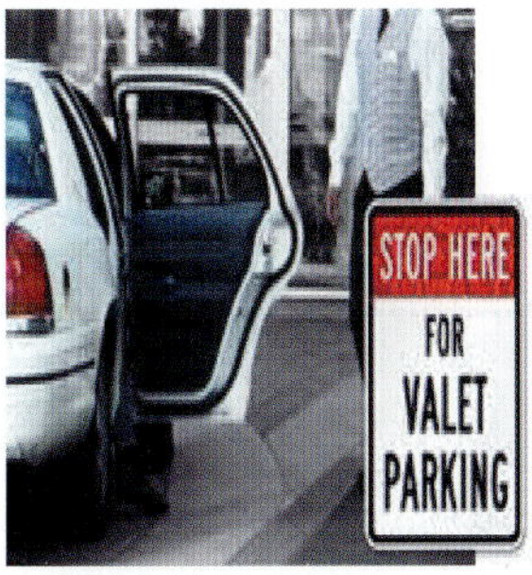


Free valet parking is available to patients and visitors to the University Hospital.
Simply follow the signs to the valet area as you enter the hospital driveway and you will be greeted by one of our friendly valet staff. Wheel chairs and other assistance are available for patients and visitors with special needs. Tipping of valet staff is not accepted. Our free valet service is available to all patients and visitors, Mon. – Fri. 7 a.m. to 6 p.m. To contact valet services please call: 585-1768.

### Words

* Valet Parking: 주차대행 서비스

* Free valet parking: 무료 주차대행 서비스

* valet staff: 주차대행 서비스 주차요원

* with special needs: 특별한 도움을 필요로 하는

* Tipping of valet staff: 주차요원들에게 팁을 주는 것

# Dialogue 2

**Patient:** Is valet parking service available here?

**Parking Attendant**: Yes, it is. Do you want to use the valet parking service?

**Patient:** Sure. What's the procedure?

**Parking Attendant**: Just hand me your key, please.

**Patient:** Um. Do you charge for the valet parking service?

**Parking Attendant:** No, we don't.

It's a courtesy service for all patients and visitors.

## Words

* What's the procedure?: 어떻게 해야 되지요?

* hand me your key: 열쇠를 제게 주시면 됩니다

* Do you charge for: ~에 이용료가 부과됩니까?

* Courtesy: 무료제공

* Courtesy phone: (공공기관 등에 설치된) 무료로 제공되는 전화서비스.

**Review:** 각각의 구문을 영작하세요.
정답은 전 페이지의 Dialogue를 참고하세요.

## Dialogue 2

**Patient:** 주차대행 서비스도 되나요?

( )

**Parking Attendant**: Yes, it is. Do you want to use the valet parking service?

**Patient:** Sure. 어떻게 해야 되지요?

( )

**Parking Attendant**: 고객님의 자동차 열쇠를 제게 주시면 됩니다.

( )

**Patient:** Um. 주차대행 서비스 이용료가 부과됩니까?

( )

**Parking Attendant:** No, we don't. 모든 환자분과 방문객을 위해 무료로 제공되는 서비스입니다.

**Drill:** 아래의 지도를 보고 각각의 질문(1-4)에 적절한 주차장을 찾아 A, B, C, D, 또는 E 로 답하세요.

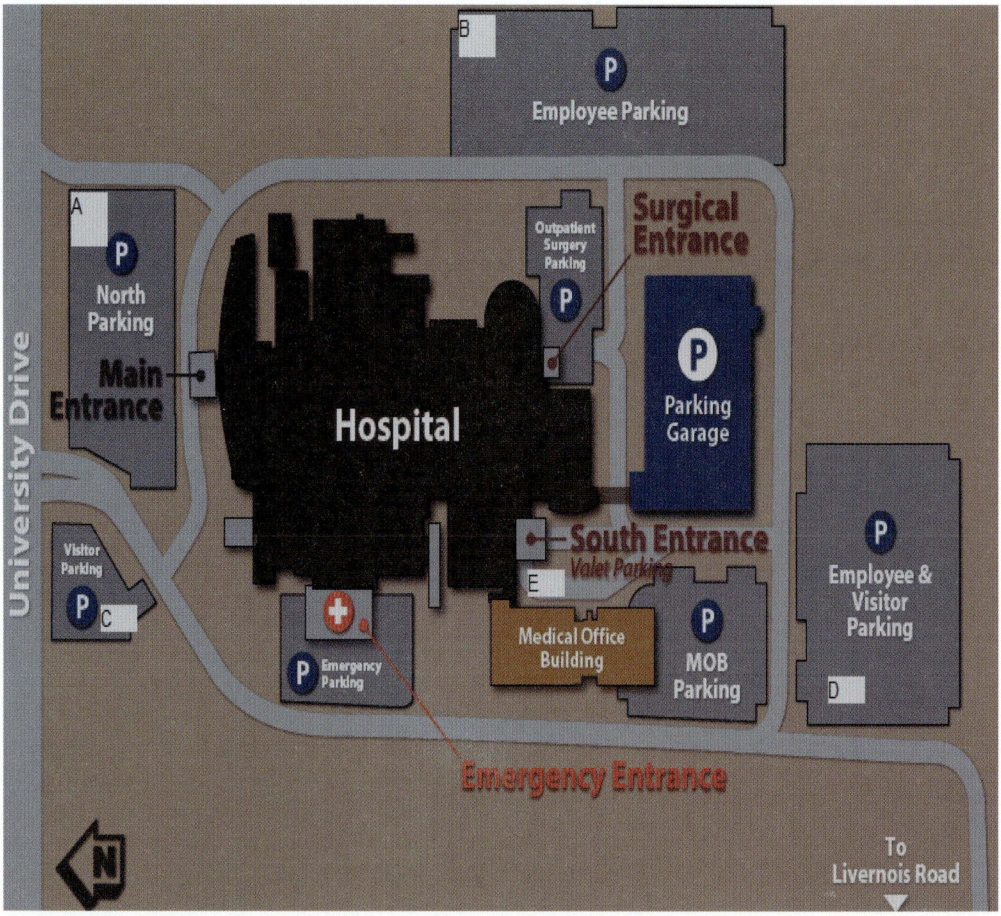


**A: North Parking, B: Employee Parking, C: Visitor Parking**
**D: Employee & Visitor Parking, E: Valet Parking**

---

## Words

* Emergency Parking: 응급실 주차장

* Outpatient Surgery Parking: 외래수술병동 주차장

* MOB (Medical Office Building) Parking: 메디컬 사무실 주차장

* Parking Garage: 주차장

1. This parking lot is located on the north side of the main hospital building, just off of University Drive. Which one is it? (     )

2. This parking area is located between South Entrance and Medical Office Building. What is the name of this parking lot? (     )

3. Hospital employees can park in these areas. Where are they? (  ,   )

4. This parking lot is located right next to MOB Parking, and both employees & visitors are allowed to park in this area. Which parking lot is it? (     )

5. How many parking lots are there in total?

## Words

* main hospital building: 병원본관

* Hospital employees: 병원 직원들

* in total: 총 몇 개

* Parking garage/Parking lot/Parking terrace: 주차공간

## 8. 정답 및 해석

## 1. 병원 안내 데스크

우리는 당신이 대학병원에서 최상의 진료를 받기를 원합니다.

만일 진료에 관한 질문이 있다면 주치의나 간호사분과 상담하세요.

또한 당신을 돕기 위한 고객서비스 팀도 있습니다.

고객 서비스팀은 당신의 질문사항을 해결해 주기 위해 도울 것입니다.

고객서비스 팀은 또한, 타지역에서 오신 분들을 위해 통역서비스, 복사, 팩스, 전화사용, 주차대행 서비스와 의전 서비스를 제공합니다.

고객서비스팀은 안내데스크, 또는 스타벅스 옆의 고객서비스 사무실에 있습니다. 또는 (801) 567-2345로 전화주세요.

## 2. 유타대학병원으로 가는 길

I-15고속도로 북쪽 방향

❶ 600 South 출구로 나가서 동쪽으로 약 2mile을 가시면 700 East가 나옵니다.

❷ 그곳에서 좌회전하여 100 South에 도달할 때까지 약 5 블럭을 가세요.

❸ 그리고, 우회전한 후 100 South를 타고 동쪽으로 1 mile을 가세요.

❹ 유타대학 캠퍼스에 도달하면 100 South가 North Campus Drive로 명칭이 바뀝니다.

❺ North Campus Drive를 타고 1mile을 더 가시면, 유타대학병원은 50 North Medical Drive거리의 오른쪽에 위치해 있습니다.

### Highway shield, 고속도로 노선번호가 삽입된 방패문양

고속도로의 방패문양은 숫자를 방패모양에 넣어 고속도로의 번호를 나타냅니다. I-15 는 캘리포니아, 네바다, 애리조나, 유타, 아이다호 및 몬타나 주를 통과하는 미국에서 4 번째로 긴 남북을 가로지르는 고속도로입니다.

## 3. 병원으로 가는 길 안내에 필요한 주요구문

### A. "~로 가는 길을 알려주시겠습니까?"

**연습문제:** 알맞은 어휘를 아래의 Words Box에서 찾아 문장을 완성하세요.

### 정답

**화장실**이 어디 있는지 말해 주실래요?

Could you tell me where the restroom is, please?

**응급실**이 어디 있는지 말해 주실래요?

Could you tell me the way to the ER (Emergency Room), please?

**접수처**가 어딘지 물어봐도 되겠어요?

May I ask you the way to the Registration Desk, please?

**안내데스크**가 어디에 있는지 알려주시겠습니까?

May I ask you how to get to the Information Desk, please?

**퇴원계**는 어디로 가는지 말해 주시겠습니까?

Can you tell me how to get to the Discharge Department, please?

**약국**으로 가는 길을 안내해 주시겠어요?

Could you show me the way to the pharmacy, please?

중환자실로 가는 길을 안내 해 주시겠어요?
Could you direct me to the ICU (Intensive Care Unit), please?

건강검진센터로 어떻게 갑니까?
How can I get to the Medical Checkup Center, please?

이 방향이 수술실로 가는 길 맞습니까?
Is this the right way to the OR (Operating Room)?

## 대화 1

**Receptionist:** 도와드릴까요?

**Patient:** 예, 저는 Dr. Park의 진료실을 찾고 있습니다.

Dr. Park과 3시에 진료예약이 있습니다.

Dr. Park의 진료실이 어디에 있는지 알려 주시겠습니까?

**Receptionist:** 예, 그런데 저도 같은 방향으로 갑니다.

제가 안내해 드리겠습니다.

저를 따라오세요.

**Patient:** 와, 감사합니다.

## B. 오른쪽 방향에 관한 표현법

**복습: 아래의 빈칸에 적합한 어휘를 넣어 문장을 완성하세요.**

**Answer: 정답**

이 복도를 따라가다 **오른쪽으로 돌아가요?**

Follow this hallway then turn right?

**모퉁이에서** 우회전 하세요.

Make a right at the corner.

**신호등에서** 우회전 하세요.

Make a right turn at the traffic light.

**2블록을 더 가서** Avon Road에 도착하면 그 곳에서 우회전 하세요.

Go two more blocks to Avon Road and turn right on **Avon Road**.

**그것은 오른쪽에 있습니다.**

It's on the right.

CK**성형외과**는 신흥은행을 막 지나면 당신의 오른쪽 방향에 있습니다.

CK Plastic Surgery Clinic will be on your right just past Shin-Heung Bank.

## C. 왼쪽 방향에 관한 표현법

**복습**

**각 문장을 영작하세요.**

**정답**

**엘리베이터에서 내려 왼쪽 방향으로 가세요.**

Turn left out of the elevator.

똑바로 두 블록 가셔서 **모퉁이에서 좌회전 하세요.**

Go straight two blocks and make a left turn at the corner.

Rochester Road에서 **좌회전 하세요.**

Turn left on Rochester Road.

약국은 **이 복도의 왼쪽에** 있습니다.

The Pharmacy is on the left of this hallway.

**엑스레이 검사실은 당신의 왼편에** 있습니다.

You'll see the X-Ray room on your left side.

**대화 2**

**Visitor:** 실례합니다. 혈액검사실이 근처에 있다고 들었는데요.

혹시 어딘지 알고 계신가요?

**A staff member:** 물론이지요. 엘리베이터를 타고 1층에서 내려서 왼쪽으로 가세요. 그리고, 복도 끝까지 가세요.

혈액검사실은 오른쪽에 있습니다. 화장실 바로 옆에 있습니다.

바로 찾으실 거예요.

**Visitor:** 감사합니다.

**A staff member:** 천만에요.

## D. 똑 바로 가세요.

### 대화 3

**Visitor:** 실례지만 서울 국제 병원은 어디에 있습니까?

**Local:** 음. 이 길을 따라 똑바로 두 블록을 가셔서 모퉁이에서 좌회전 하세요. 그러면 커다란 파란색 건물이 보입니다.

바로 그 건물입니다. 쉽게 찾으실 겁니다.

**Visitor:** 감사합니다.

**Local:** 천만에요.

## E. 계단을 이용하세요

### 대화 4

**Visitor:** 세포병리실을 찾고 있습니다.

어디에 있는지 알려주시겠습니까?

**Receptionist:** 예. 삼층에 있어요.

우선, 계단이 나올 때까지 이 복도를 따라 가세요.

여기가 이층이니 3층으로 가시기 위해 계단 두 층을 올라 가세요.

세포병리실 입구가 보일 것입니다.

쉽게 찾을 것입니다.

**Visitor:** 정말 고맙습니다.

## F. 엘리베이터를 이용하세요

### 대화 5

**Patient:** 이비인후과가 어디에 있는지 혹시 알고 계십니까?

**Receptionist:** 예. 엘리베이터를 타고 3층으로 올라가세요.

엘리베이터에서 내려서 왼쪽으로 가세요.

당신의 오른쪽에서 두 번째 방입니다.

**Patient:** 알겠습니다. 3층에 있지요, 그렇지요?

**Receptionist:** 맞아요. 3층에 있어요.

**Patient:** 알겠습니다. 감사합니다.

**Receptionist:** 천만에요.

## G. 에스컬레이터를 이용하세요

### 대화 6

**Receptionist:** 도와 드릴까요?

**Visitor:** 예. 스타벅스가 어디에 있는지 알려 주시겠습니까?

**Receptionist:** 물론이죠. 로비에 있습니다.

에스컬레이터를 타고 한층 내려가셔서 오른쪽으로 가세요.

그런 후, 안내데스크로 가세요.

스타벅스는 안내데스크 바로 옆에 있습니다.

**Visitor:** 감사합니다.

**Receptionist:** 천만에요.

## H. 이 복도를 따라가세요.

### 대화 7

**Visitor:** 저는 소아심장센터를 찾고 있습니다.

혹시 어디에 있는지 아시나요?

**A staff member:** 예. 이 복도를 따라가세요.

복도 끝에 도달하면 왼쪽으로 가세요.

그러면, 소아심장센터는 왼쪽에서 두 번째 방입니다.

**Visitor:** 미안하지만, 이해가 안됐어요. 다시 한번 말씀해 주시겠어요?

**A staff member:** 물론이죠. 이 복도 끝까지 따라가세요.

그리고 왼쪽으로 가세요.

**Visitor:** 이 복도를 끝까지 따라가다가 왼쪽으로 가요?

**A staff member:** 맞습니다.

소아심장센터는 왼쪽에서 두 번째 방입니다.

**Visitor:** 알겠습니다. 정말 감사합니다.

**A staff member:** 천만에요.

## 대화 8

**Visitor:** 실례합니다.

저는 엘리베이터를 찾고 있습니다.

이 근처에 엘리베이터가 있나요?

**John Doe:** 예. 저쪽 끝에 있어요.

복도 끝까지 따라 가셔서 왼쪽으로 가세요. 그러면 방문객 전용 엘리베이터가 보입니다.

**Visitor:** 복도 끝까지 가는 것 맞지요?

**John Doe:** 네.

**Visitor:** 감사합니다.

**John Doe:** 천만에요.

## I. ~을 지나가다

### 대화 9

**Visitor:** 실례합니다.

메디컬 플라자에 어떻게 가야 하나요?

**Local:** 우체국에 도착할 때까지 이 길을 따라 계속 가세요.

그리고, 우체국에서 좌회전 하세요.

**Visitor:** 알겠습니다.

**Local:** 좌회전한 후에, 도서관을 지나세요.

그러면 도서관 바로 옆 건물이에요.

**Visitor:** 여기에서 먼가요?

**Local:** 그렇지 않아요.

**Visitor:** 알겠습니다. 감사합니다.

**Local:** 천만에요.

**대화 10**

**Patient:** 영상의학과가 어디에 있는지 말씀해 주시겠습니까?

**Receptionist:** 예, 응급실을 지날 때까지 계속 가세요. 그러면 영상의학과가 응급실 바로 옆에 있는 것을 보시게 될 것입니다.

**Patient:** 알겠습니다. 감사합니다.

**Receptionist:** 천만에요.

## J. ~뒤에/~앞에

### 대화 11

**Patient:** 실례합니다.

진료상담실이 어디에 있는지 아십니까?

**Nurse:** 예. 진료실 앞에 있습니다.

**Patient:** 감사합니다.

그리고 가장 가까운 은행도 알려 주시겠습니까?

**Nurse:** 물론이죠. 본관 뒤에 있습니다.

## K. ~의 모퉁이에

### 대화 12

**Visitor:** 강동경희대학교 국제의료센터로 가는 방법을 알려주시겠습니까?
**Jane Doe:** 물론이죠.

**Visitor:** 여기에서 먼가요?
**Jane Doe:** 아니요. 이 길을 따라 두 블록을 더 가세요. 그리고 좌회전 하세요.
그러면 강동경희대병원 국제 클리닉센터는 길 모퉁이에 있을 것입니다.

**Visitor:** 감사합니다.
**Jane Doe:** 천만에요.

## L. 대각선방향에서

의미: 마치 사각형의 한 모퉁이에 서 있는 것처럼 지금 현 위치에서 대각선 방향에 있습니다.
"4-H센터에서 대각선 방향에 집 한 채가 있습니다."

### 대화 13

**Visitor:** 우체국은 어디에 있나요?

**John Doe:** 이 건물에서 대각선 방향에 있습니다.

### 대화 14

**Jane Doe:** 이 근처에 있는 어린이책 서점을 알려주시겠습니까?

**Local:** 물론이죠. 어린이책 서점은 아담스 에비뉴에 있는 도서관의 대각선 방향에 위치해 있습니다.

## Chapter 2

**Drill: 아래의 글을 읽고 Bank of America의 위치를 그리세요.**

**정답**

재활센터는 처치빌 로드와 메인 스트릿의 모퉁이에 있습니다.

아메리카은행은 재활센터에서 대각선방향에 위치해 있습니다.

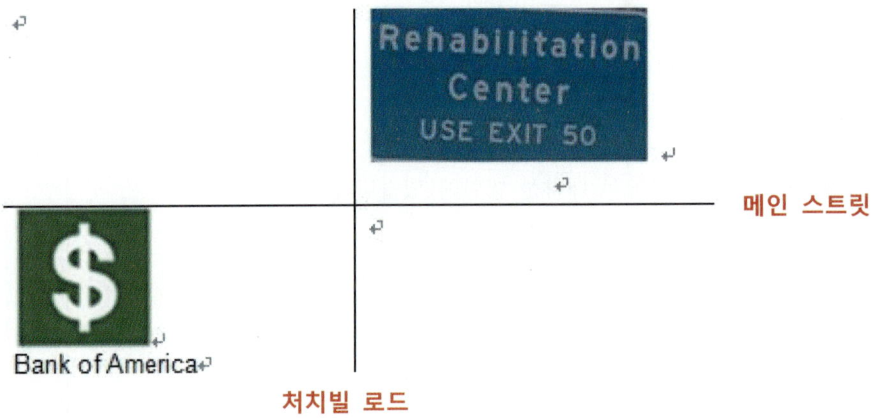

## 4. 연습문제

오레곤주의 포틀랜드시에서 시계건전지 교체, 손목시계와 시계수리, 복원과 보석 수리를 가장 잘하는 곳입니다.

우리의 상점은 Laurel Wood거리와 Beaverton-Hillsdale거리의 모퉁이에 있고 US 은행에서 대각선 방향에 있습니다.

**정답: 8108이 쓰여진 상점 입니다.**

**연습문제**

**정답:**

* Make us your first and last stop for all of your medical supply needs:

의료제품에 관한 모든 것을 판매하며 최고의 서비스를 제공하는 곳입니다.

Chapter 2

## 5. 주요구문

### 연습문제: 다음의 질문을 영작하세요.

### 정답

A1: It's **in front of** the pharmacy.

A2: **There's one** on the University Street.

A3. I'm looking for **a dermatology department.**

A4. **Rehabilitation center** is **across the street.**

A5. Could you tell me **the shortest route** to get to LK Korean Medicine Clinic?

A6. Where is **the entrance to the Outpatient Clinic**?

A7. Could you tell me where **the Inpatient Ward** is?

A8. Which room is it in **the surgical ward**?

A9. It's **in the middle of the hallway.**

A10. You need to walk down to **the third door and turn right.**

A11: Could you tell me where I can take **the subway line number 3**?

A 12: You need to get off at the Jamsil Station and then **go out the Exit number 10.**

## 6. 병원시설 업무시간과 병원진료시간

### 식당가

#### 구내식당

**Level A** 에 위치함. 아침, 점심, 저녁 식사.

구내식당 영업시간: 월요일부터 금요일까지는 오전 6:30-오후 10:00

토요일, 일요일, 그리고 공휴일은 오전 8:00-오후 8:00

**대화 1**

**Receptionist:** 카페테리아입니다. 무엇을 도와 드릴까요?

**Customer:** 영업시간이 어떻게 되나요?

**Receptionist:** 월요일부터 금요일까지는 오전 6:30부터 오후 10:00까지 문을 열니다.

토요일, 일요일, 그리고 공휴일에는 오전 8:00에서 오후 8:00까지 문을 엽니다. 또 다른 질문 사항이 있으십니까?

**Customer:** 아니요. 감사합니다.

**Chapter 2**

## 스타벅스

로비근처 Level 1 에 위치함

영업시간: 하루 24시간 주 7일

### 대화 2

**Receptionist:** 스타벅스 입니다. 무엇을 도와드릴까요?

**Visitor:** 예. 영업시간을 알고 싶은데요.

**Receptionist:** 알려드리겠습니다. 우리는 하루 24시간 주 7일 열고 있습니다. 고객님을 위하여 언제나 열고 있습니다.

**Visitor:** 와, 연중 무휴이군요. 그렇지요?

**Receptionist:** 예, 그렇습니다. 다른 문의 사항이 있습니까?

**Visitor:** 예. 위치가 어떻게 되지요?

**Receptionist:** 우리는 Level 1 의 로비 근처에 위치해 있습니다.

**Visitor:** 알겠습니다. 곧 들르겠습니다.

**Receptionist:** 네, 곧 뵙겠습니다.

## 베타 클리닉 진료시간

베타 클리닉 진료시간: 월-금 오전 8시-오후 4시

클리닉은 예약제로도 진료를 받고 또는 예약 없이도 진료를 받을 수 있습니다.

예약하실 때 전화 번호: 476-8976

### 대화 3

**Patient:** 진료시간이 어떻게 되지요?

**Receptionist:** 우리의 진료시간은 월요일부터 금요일, 오전 8시부터 오후 4시입니다. 저희 클리닉과 예약을 하셨나요?

**Patient:** 아닙니다. 하지만 진료를 보기 위해 예약을 하고 싶습니다.

**Receptionist:** 그러시면, 이 번호로 전화를 하셔서 예약을 하세요. 번호는 476-8976 입니다.

**Patient:** 감사합니다.

**Receptionist:** 천만에요.

Chapter 2

## 연습문제

### 정답

1. American Fork Hospital
2. UCHD, Orem, Payson and Saratoga
3. Wednesday-UCHD, Tuesday-Payson City Center
4. None
5. 851-7025

## 안내도(층별 안내도)

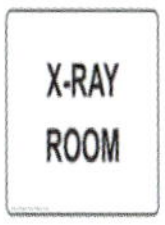


**Patient:** 엑스레이 검사실이 어디에 있는지 알려 주시겠습니까?
**Receptionist:** 예. 먼저, 이 복도 끝까지 가세요. 그러면, 엑스레이 검사실이 응급실 바로 옆에 있습니다.

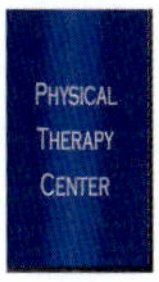


**Patient:** 실례합니다. 물리 치료실이 어디에 있는지 말씀해 주시겠습니까?
**Receptionist:** 물론이죠. 장애우 전용 입구에서 두 계단 밑으로 내려가세요. 그러면, 왼쪽에서 두 번째 방입니다.
쉽게 찾으실 거예요.

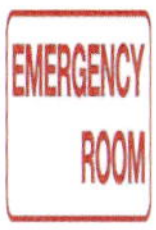


**Patient:** 응급실로 가는 길을 알려주시겠습니까?

**Receptionist:** 알겠습니다. 응급실은 1층에 있습니다. CT스캔실 바로 옆에 있습니다.

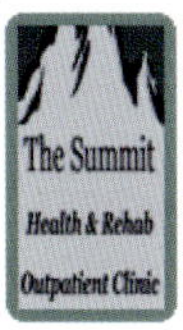


**Patient:** 외래진료소를 어떻게 가야 하나요?
**Receptionist:** 외래진료소는 2층에 위치해 있습니다.
엘리베이터를 타고 2층에서 내리세요. 엘리베이터에서 내려서 왼쪽으로 가신 후 바닥의 노란색 화살표를 따라가세요.

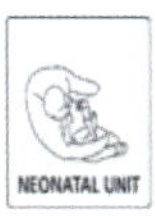


**Patient:** 신생아실은 어디에 있습니까?
**Receptionist:** 3층에 있습니다. 분만실 건너편에 있어요.

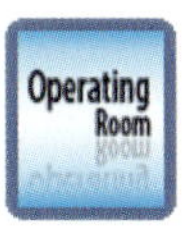


**Patient:** 수술실이 가까운 곳에 있나요?
**Receptionist:** 예. 3층에 있습니다. 중환자실 바로 건너편에 있어요.

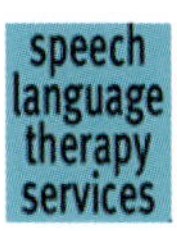


**Patient:** 혹시 언어치료실이 어디에 있는지 알려 주시겠습니까?
**Receptionist:** 물리치료실 바로 옆방입니다.

### 대화 4

**Receptionist:** 무엇을 도와드릴까요?

**Visitor:** 헌츠먼 암 연구소를 찾고 있습니다.

**Receptionist:** 알겠습니다. 방문객 전용 엘리베이터를 타고 3층으로 가세요. 그런 다음 엘리베이터에서 내려서 오른쪽으로 가세요. 임상 신경과학 센터를 지날 때까지 계속 가세요.
그러면, 헌츠먼 암 연구소는 당신의 왼쪽에 있을 것입니다.
이해가 되십니까?

**Visitor:** 죄송합니다만, 이해가 잘 안돼요. 다시 말씀해 주시겠습니까?

**Receptionist:** 물론이죠. 우선, 방문객 전용 엘리베이터를 타고 3층으로 가세요.

**Visitor:** 음. 방문객 전용 엘리베이터는 어디에 있나요?

**Receptionist:** 로비에 있는 스타벅스 바로 옆에 있어요.

**Visitor:** 로비에 있는 스타벅스 바로 옆에 있는 방문객 전용 엘리베이터를 타고 3층에서 내리는 거죠. 그렇지요?

**Receptionist:** 맞습니다. 그 다음에는, 임상 신경과학 센터를 지날 때까지 복도를 쭉 따라 가세요. 그러면, 당신의 왼편에 헌츠먼 암 연구소를 보실 수 있습니다. 금방 찾으실 것입니다.

**Visitor:** 알겠습니다.
임상 신경과학 센터에 도착할 때까지 복도를 쭉 따라 가는 거지요. 그러면, 헌츠먼 암 연구소가 나의 왼편에 있는 것 맞지요?

**Receptionist:** 맞아요.

**Visitor:** 정말 감사합니다.

## 7. 주차안내

### 자가주차

만일 본인이 직접 주차하기를 원한다면, 병원으로 향하는 길 오른쪽에 위치해 있는 환자 및 방문객전용 주차장에 무료주차를 하실 수 있습니다.
주차를 하신 장소와 병원의 어느 출입문을 사용하셨는지 꼭 기억하세요.

**대화 1**

**Visitor:** 실례합니다. 이 근처에 주차장이 있나요?

**Local:** 예, 병원 진입로 근처에 있습니다.

**Visitor:** 찾기가 어려운가요? 제가 이곳을 처음 방문해서요.

**Local:** 어렵지 않습니다. 주차장으로 가는 표식이 있습니다.

실은 표식은 바로 앞에 있습니다.

표식을 따라가세요. 어렵지 않습니다.

**Visitor:** 그런데, 주차비는 무료입니까?

**Local:** 예, 무료입니다.

**Visitor:** 알겠습니다. 감사합니다.

## 주차대행 서비스

대학병원에 오신 환자와 방문객은 주차대행 서비스를 무료로 이용할 수 있습니다. 병원으로 진입하는 길에 들어서서 주차대행 서비스로 향하는 표시를 따라가시면 우리의 친절한 주차대행 서비스 주차요원이 여러분을 맞이할 것입니다. 특별한 도움을 필요로 하는 환자 또는 방문객을 위해 휠체어와 다른 도움 장비가 제공됩니다. 주차대행 서비스 주차요원들은 팁을 받지 않습니다.

우리의 무료 주차대행 서비스는 월요일-금요일, 오전 7시에서 오후 6시까지 모든 환자와 방문객들에게 제공됩니다. 주차대행 서비스 관련 문의 사항은 585-1768로 전화 주세요.

### 대화 2

**Patient:** 주차대행 서비스도 되나요?

**Parking Attendant**: 예, 됩니다. 주차대행 서비스를 이용하시겠습니까?

**Patient:** 물론입니다. 어떻게 해야 되지요?

**Parking Attendant**: 고객님의 자동차 열쇠를 제게 주시면 됩니다.

**Patient:** 음. 주차대행 서비스 이용료가 부과됩니까?

**Parking Attendant:** 아닙니다. 모든 환자분과 방문객을 위해 무료로 제공되는 서비스입니다.

**연습문제:** 아래의 지도를 보고 각각의 질문(1-4)에 적절한 주차장을 찾아 A, B, C, D 또는 E 로 답하세요.

1. University Drive를 막 벗어났을 때, 이 주차장은 병원본관의 북쪽에 위치해 있습니다. 어느 주차장인가요? (   )

2. 이 주차장은 South Entrance 와 Medical Office Building 사이에 위치해 있습니다. 이 주차장의 이름은 무엇입니까? (      )

3. 병원 직원들이 이곳에 주차를 할 수 있습니다. 어디인가요? ( ,   )

4. 이 주차장은 MOB 주차장 바로 옆에 있습니다. 그리고 이 곳에는 직원과 방문객 모두 주차할 수 있습니다. 어느 주차장입니까? (    )

5. 주차장은 총 몇 개입니까? (      )

정답: 1. (A), 2. (E, Valet Parking), 3. (B, D), 4. (D), 5. (9)

# Chapter 3

# Doctor's Fee

# 진료비

## 1. Key Words for Doctor's Fee
진료비 관련 주요어휘

- **Words to know, 어휘**
- **What is plastic money? 플라스틱화폐란?**
- **Words, 어휘**

# Words to know

The bill,

List of charges: 청구서

Doctor's bill,

Doctor's fee,

Doctor's consultation fee,

A consultation fee: 진료비

Medical expenses: 의료비용

Medical coverage: 보험이 적용되는 의료비(의료급여)

Payment Method: 지불방법

Cashier: 수납원

Receipt: 영수증

Deposit: 보증금

* Big Deposit: 전세보증금

Bank Account Number: 은행계좌 번호

Bank's Physical Address: 은행 주소

Bank Wire: 타 은행으로 송금

# What is plastic money?

## Do you accept plastic money?

Plastic money is the alternative to the cash or the standard 'money'. Plastic money is used to refer to the credit cards or the debit cards that we use to make purchases in our everyday life.

**Debit card**

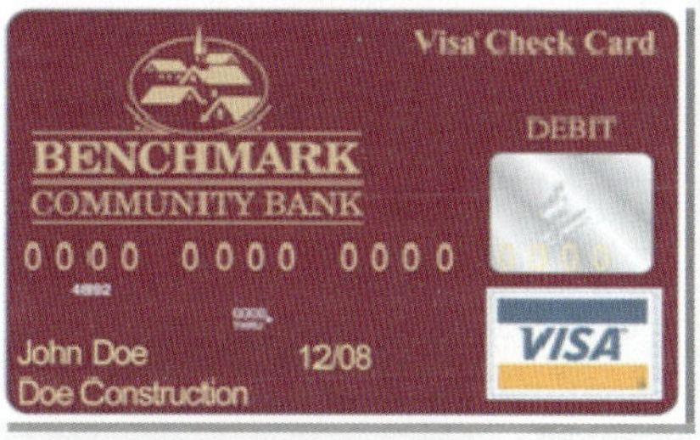


**Vs**

**Credit card**

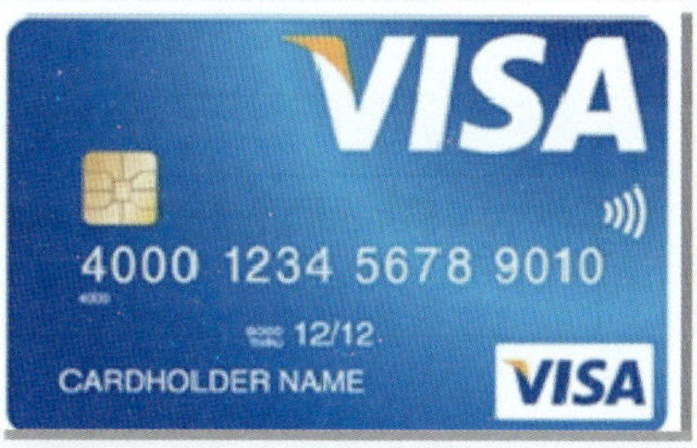

## Words

* John Doe: 홍길동

* CARDHOLDER NAME: 카드 소유자 성명

* accept: (지불방법으로) 신용카드를 받습니다.

* plastic money: 신용카드 또는 직불카드를 총칭함.

* Credit card: 신용카드

* Debit card/Check card: 직불카드

* alternative to: ~을 대신하는

* standard 'money': 기존의 '화폐'

* purchase: 구매하다

## 2. Hospitalized Foreign Patient without Health Insurance
의료보험이 없는 외국인 입원 환자의 경우

- **Dialogue, 대화**
- **Words, 어휘**
- **Review, 복습**

# Dialogue 1

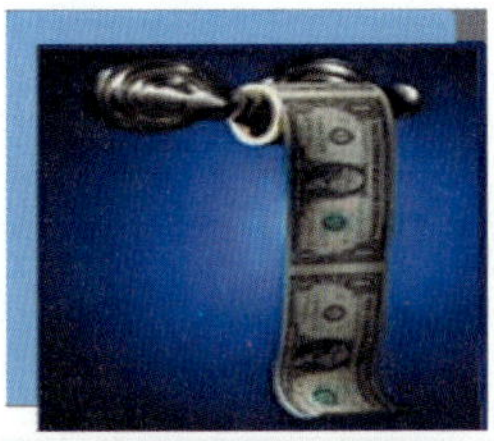

**Receptionist:** How are you planning to pay for your medical expenses? Are you under any medical insurance?

**Patient:** No, I'm not. I'd like to pay the bill myself.

**Receptionist:** I see. If you are not covered by any health insurance, you need to leave a deposit please.

**Patient:** How much should I leave for the deposit?

**Receptionist**: You need to leave half of your medical expenses, please. Also, you need to pay the rest of your medical expenses at the time of discharge.

**Patient:** Okay. Do you accept credit cards?

**Receptionist:** Yes. We accept VISA card.

**Patient:** Then, I will pay it with my VISA card.
By the way, how much is the charge for the blood test?

**Receptionist:** It is 100 dollars.

**Patient:** Okay. How much does it all come to?

**Receptionist:** With your deposit, the total comes to 1,500 dollars.

**Patient:** I see. Here is my VISA card.

**Receptionist:** Alright. Then, I will charge it on your VISA card.

## Words

* medical expenses: 병원비

* pay the bill myself: 자비로 지불하다

* I will pay the bill with cash.: 현찰로 지불하겠습니다.

* deposit: 보증금

* half of: ~(금액)의 반

* at the time of discharge: 퇴원하시는 날에

* 총 얼마를 지불해야 하나요?

  How much do I owe you in all?

  How much does it all come to?

  How much is it all together?

  How much is it in total?

* blood test: 혈액검사

* charge it on your VISA card: 비자카드로 결제해 드리겠습니다

**Review:** 괄호 안의 구문을 번호에 맞게 영작하세요.
정답은 전 페이지의 Dialogue를 참고하세요.

**Dialogue: Hospitalized Foreign Patient without Health Insurance**

①: 병원비 ②: 의료보험 ③: 자비로 지불할 것입니다
④: 보증금을 내셔야 합니다 ⑤: 의료비의 반액을
⑥: 나머지 반액은 ⑦: 신용카드도 받으시나요

**Receptionist:** How are you planning to pay for your (① ).

Are you under any (② ).

**Patient:** No, I'm not. I'd like to (③ ).

**Receptionist:** I see. If you are not covered by any health insurance, you need to (④ ), please.

**Patient:** How much should I leave for the deposit?

**Receptionist**: You need to leave (⑤ ) please.

Also, you need to pay (⑥ ) at the time of discharge.

**Patient:** Okay. Do you (⑦ )?

⑧: 비자카드로 지불하겠습니다.
⑨: 총 얼마를 지불해야 하나요?
⑩: 보증금과 합해서

**Receptionist:** Yes. We accept VISA card.

**Patient:** Then, I will (⑧ ).

By the way, how much is the charge for the blood test?

**Receptionist:** It is 100 dollars.

**Patient:** Okay. (⑨ )?

**Receptionist:** (⑩ ), the total comes to 1,500 dollars.

**Patient:** I see. Here is my VISA card.

**Receptionist:** Alright. Then, I will charge it on your VISA card.

## 3. Key Expressions
주요구문

- **Drill, 연습문제**

**Drill: 상자 안에 나열된 단어를 아래의 문장에 넣어 주요구문을 완성하세요.**

| | |
|---|---|
| registration desk | consultation room |
| medical insurance | waiting ticket |
| health insurance certificate | cost |
| registration form | health insurance |
| consultation | medical insurance form |
| fee | blood test |
| doctor's examination room | purchased |

**접수 창구**는 어디에 있습니까?

Where's the ________, please?

**접수 용지**를 어디 가면 얻을 수 있을까요?

Where can I get a ________ ?

그녀의 **순서대기표**는 17번입니다.

She has a ________ number 17.

## Chapter 3

**<u>의료보험</u>**이 있습니까? (같은 답을 두 번 써도 됩니다.)

Do you have [          ] ?

Are you covered under [          ] ?

Are you covered by any [          ] ?

이것이 저의 **<u>의료보험증서</u>**입니다.

Here's my [          ] .

**<u>의료보험 양식</u>**은 여기에 제출해야 합니까?

Do I need to submit my [          ] here?

한국에 오기 전에 의료보험에 **<u>가입</u>**하셨습니까?

Have you [          ] medical insurance before coming to Korea?

**<u>진찰료</u>**는 얼마이지요?

What's the [          ] please?

**<u>진료상담비</u>**는 얼마인가요?

How much do you charge for a [          ] ?

이 **<u>혈액검사</u>** 비용은 얼마입니까?

How much do you charge for the [          ] ?

**비용은** 얼마 되지 않습니다.

It won't [          ] much.

**진료실**은 어디 있어요?

Where's the [          ] please?

**진료상담실**은 어디 있어요?

Where's the [          ] please?

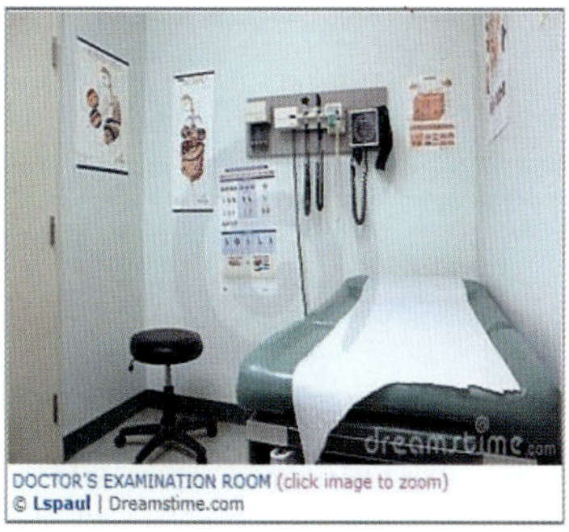


**A Doctor's Examination Room:**
**진료실**

vs

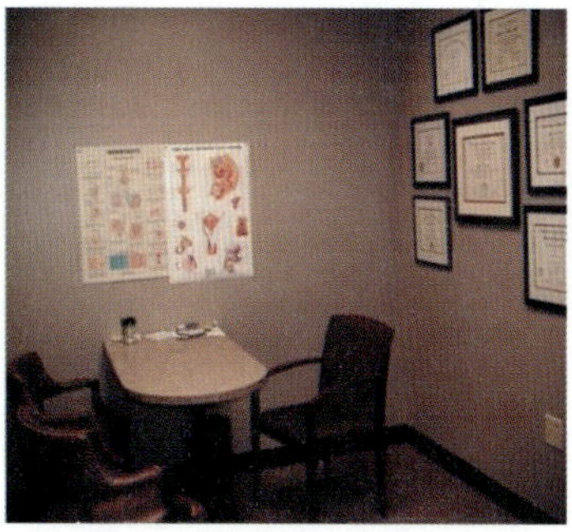

**A Consultation Room:**
**진료 상담실**

## 4. With International Health Insurance,
해외의료보험이 있는 경우

- **Words to know, 어휘**
- **Medical and Dental Insurance Cards, 의료보험과 치과보험카드**
- ***Code breaker's corner: 로리와 함께 하는 미국문화 엿보기***
    - **Personal Check: 개인수표**
    - **Drill: Let's write a personal check!! 개인수표 작성해보기!**
- **Medical Certificate, 진단서**
- **Co-payment, 공동부담금**

# Words to know

**Medical insurance:** 의료보험

**Medical insurance subscriber:** 의료보험 가입자

**Beneficiaries of medical insurance:** 의료보험 혜택자

**Effective date:** 효력 발생 날짜

**Name of provider making charge:** 보험회사에 진료행위를 청구하는 의사분의 성명

**Medical certificate:** 진단서

**Payee:** 보험료 수령자

**Policy or identification number of coverage:** 보험 증서 번호

**Type of provider:** 진료받은 진료과목 의사 선생님

(예: Plastic surgeon, 성형외과 의사선생님)

**Date of service or purchase:** 의료보험 카드로 진료 받은 날짜

**International medical claim form:** 해외 진료 청구서

**Co-payment:** 공동부담금

Chapter 3

# Medical and Dental Insurance Cards

제가 미국에서 사용한 의료보험카드입니다.

보험회사는 블루크로스 블루쉴드입니다.

**Medical Insurance Card:** 의료보험카드

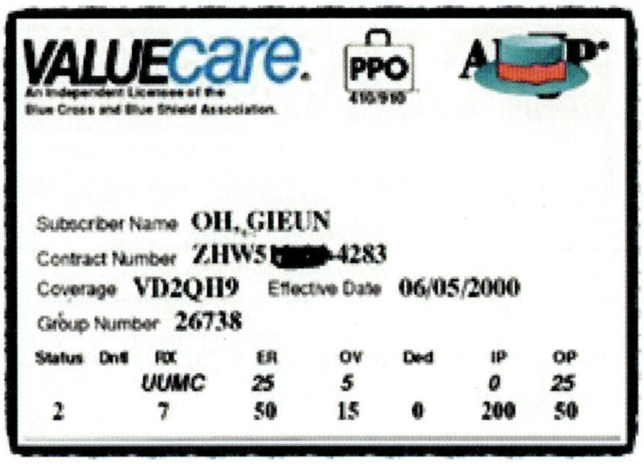


**Dental Insurance Card:** 치과의료보험카드

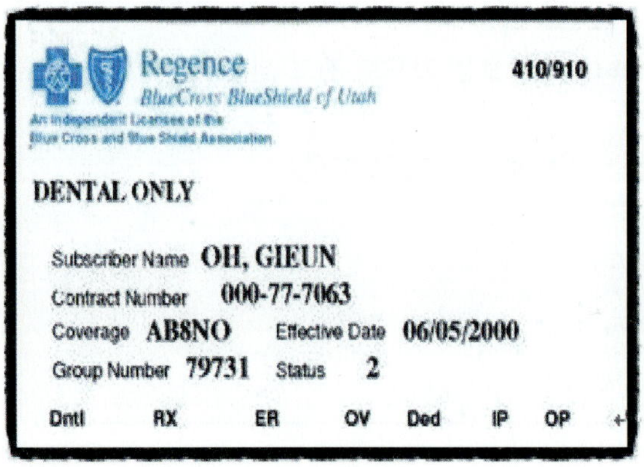

## *Code breaker's corner: 로리와 함께 하는 미국문화 엿보기*

### Personal Check: 개인수표

### Drill: Let's write a personal check!! 개인수표 작성해보기!

각각의 해당 난에 본인의 이름 및 주소, 거래은행의 이름 및 주소를 적으시고, 구매한 물건의 가격, 가격을 지불한 대상, 구매당일 날짜, 서명 및 간단한 메모를 영어로 기입하세요.

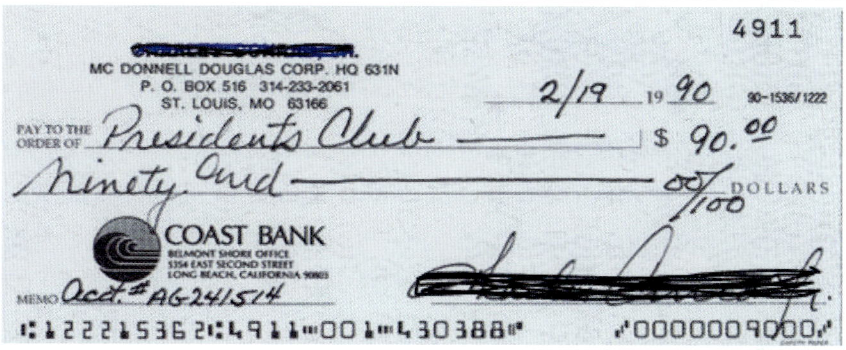
4911
MC DONNELL DOUGLAS CORP. HQ 631N
P. O. BOX 516 314-233-2061
ST. LOUIS, MO 63166
2/19 19 90
90-1536/1222
PAY TO THE ORDER OF Presidents Club
$ 90.00
Ninety and 00/100 DOLLARS
COAST BANK
MEMO Acct.# AG-241514

개인수표를 작성한 분은 1990년 2월 19일에 프레지던트 클럽에 90달러를 지불했습니다. 구매자의 은행은 COAST BANK입니다. 메모란에는 구매자가 Acct# AG 241514를 기입했습니다.

**Name:** **117**
**Address:**
**City, State, Zip:**

**Date:** / /

**Pay to the**
**Order of**____________________________ $ ________

____________________________ ***Dollars***

**Bank Name:**
**Bank Address:**

**Memo:** ________ Signature ______________

## Words

* name: 구매자 이름

* address: 구매자의 주소

* City, State, Zip: 구매자가 사는 도시, 주, 우편번호

* Pay to the order of(=Payee): 지불 받는 대상

(물건을 구매 후 돈이 지불되는 곳/대상)

* bank name: 구매자가 거래하는 은행이름

* bank address: 구매자가 거래하는 은행주소

* Memo: 구매자가 구매한 내용, 품목에 관한 간략한 기록

* Acct =Account, (은행 등의) 계좌

* # =number, 번호

* Acct#=Account number: 계좌번호

* Signature: 구매자의 서명

# Medical Certificate

## MEDICAL CERTIFICATE

I, the undersigned Doctor in medicine, (full name)................................

..........................................................................................

certify that I have examined the blood test results and chest X-rays of Mr./Mrs.

(full name)

..........................................................................................

Nationality:..........................................................................

Passport No.:.......................................................................

Date and place of birth:......................................................

Residing at...........................................................................

and have found him/her (please check the appropriate box):

| | Free of the following Illness | Afflicted with the following illness |
|---|---|---|
| HIV/AIDS | | |
| Hepatitis B and C | | |
| Tuberculosis | | |
| Syphilis | | |

Issued at..............................................on...................................

Signature of the Doctor.......................................................

Stamps of doctor's office......................................................

## Chapter 3

---

### Words

* Medical Certificate: 진단서

* undersigned: 아래에 서명한

* certify: 증명합니다.

* Nationality: 국적

* Residing at: 거주지

* afflicted: 질병을 앓고 있는

* Hepatitis B and C: B형과 C형 간염

* Tuberculosis: 결핵

* Syphilis: 매독

* issued at: 발행기관

* Stamps of doctor's office: 병원직인

# Co-payment

**Co-payment: 공동부담금**

- 환자가 진료를 받을 때 지불하는 소액의 금액
- 진료의 경중과는 상관없이 지불하는 금액

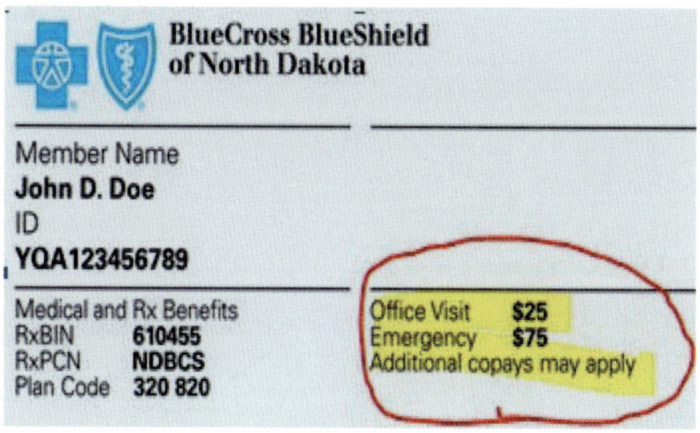


**Office Visit:** 외래진료 시는 $25를 공동부담금으로 지불합니다.

**Emergency:** 응급실 방문 시는 $75를 공동부담금으로 지불합니다.

**Additional co-pays may apply:** 추가된 공동부담금이 발생할 수 있습니다.

## 5. For Office Visit Patient with International Medical Insurance
해외보험이 있는 외래환자

- **Dialogue 2, 대화 2**
- **Words, 어휘**
- **Review, 복습**

# Dialogue 2

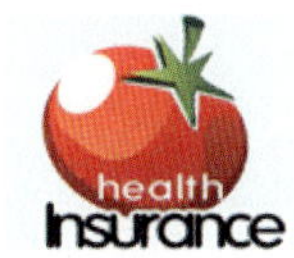


**Receptionist**: How do you plan to pay for your visit?

**Patient:** I'm covered by a foreign medical insurance company. Is it acceptable?

**Receptionist:** What is the name of your medical insurance company?

**Patient:** I am covered by BLUECROSS BLUESHIELD medical insurance.

**Receptionist**: Do you have a letter of guarantee from your insurance company?

**Patient:** Yes, I do. Here it is.

**Receptionist**: Let me see.

I need to check whether your insurance company has a direct billing arrangement with us.

**Patient:** I see.

**Receptionist:** Good news!

Your insurance company is under our direct billing arrangement.

However, you still need to pay a part of the bill such as co-payment.

**Patient:** Alright. Can I pay my co-payment with credit card?

**Receptionist:** Yes, you can.

**Patient:** How much do I owe?

**Receptionist**: Your co-payment is $30.

**Patient:** And, how much is my medical expenses in total?

**Receptionist**: Your total comes to $3,500.

**Patient**: Alright.

**Receptionist:** I'm going to ask you some questions on your medical insurance. What is your medical insurance contract number?

**Patient:** My medical insurance contract number is ANF 255-98-2364.

**Receptionist:** What is the name of the subscriber?

**Patient:** Ken Johnson.

**Receptionist:** What's your current mailing address?

**Patient:** #703 Spy Glass Apt, 3rd Ave, Salt Lake City, UT 84103.

**Receptionist:** When is the effective date of your medical insurance?

**Patient:** 09/12/95.

**Receptionist**: What's your employment status?

**Patient:** I am actively employed.

**Receptionist:** Can I make a photocopy of your medical insurance card?

**Patient:** Sure. Here is my card.

**Receptionist:** I have a Blue Card Worldwide International Claim Form for you to fill out.

**Patient:** Alright. Let me fill it out and bring it back to you.

**Receptionist:** Thank you. By the way, do you need copies of the bill and a medical certificate?

**Patient:** That's right. I might need them to claim my medical expenses when I go back to my country, just in case.

Thank you for your consideration.

## Words

* pay for your visit: 진료비를 지불하다

* letter of guarantee: 의료보험 보증서

* Direct billing arrangement (Cashless pay plan): 환자가 진료비를 병원에 직접지불하는 대신 의료 보험회사가 진료비를 환자가 진료 받은 병원에 직접 지불하는 제도.

* Co-payment: 공동부담금

* insurance contract number: 의료보험 계약번호

* the name of the subscriber: 보험가입자의 이름

* current mailing address: 현재 거주지의 주소

* effective date: 효력발생일

* employment status: 고용상태

* actively employed: 근무하고 있습니다

* make a photocopy of: ~을 복사하다.

* fill out: 작성하다

* Blue Card Worldwide International Claim Form: 블루카드 월드와이드 국제 보험청구서 양식

* copies of: 사본

* the bill: 청구서

* medical certificate: 진단서

* claim: 청구하다

* consideration: 배려

**Review:** 괄호 안에 구문을 영작하세요.
정답은 전 페이지의 Dialogue를 참고하세요.

### Dialogue 2

**Receptionist**: 진료비를 어떻게 지불하시겠습니까?
( )

**Patient:** I'm covered by a foreign medical insurance company. Is it acceptable?

**Receptionist:** What is the name of your medical insurance company?

**Patient:** I am covered by BLUECROSS BLUESHIELD medical insurance.

**Receptionist**: 의료보험회사로부터 의료보험 보증서를 받아오셨나요?
( )

**Patient:** Yes, I do. Here it is.

**Receptionist**: Let me see.
제가 고객님의 보험회사와 우리병원이 직접 청구하는 방식을 따르는지 확인해 보겠습니다.
( )

**Patient:** I see.

**Receptionist:** Good news!

Your insurance company is under our direct billing arrangement.

**하지만 고객님은 공동부담금과 같은 청구서의 일부는 지불하셔야 합니다.**

**( )**

**Patient:** Alright. Can I pay my co-payment with credit card?

**Receptionist:** Yes, you can.

**Patient:** How much do I owe?

**Receptionist**: Your co-payment is $30.

**Patient:** And, how much is my medical expenses in total?

**Receptionist**: **총 진료비는 $3,500입니다.**

**( )**

**Patient**: Alright.

**Receptionist:** I'm going to ask you some questions on your medical insurance. **의료보험 계약번호가 무엇입니까?**

**( )**

**Patient:** My medical insurance contract number is ANF 255-98-2364.

**Receptionist: 보험가입자의 이름은 무엇입니까?**

**( )**

**Patient:** Ken Johnson.

**Receptionist:** 현재 거주지의 주소는요?

( )

**Patient:** #703 Spy Glass Apt, 3rd Ave, Salt Lake City, UT 84103.

**Receptionist:** When is the effective date of your medical insurance?

**Patient:** 09/12/95.

**Receptionist**: 지금 고용상태는요?

( )

**Patient:** 직장에서 근무하고 있습니다.

( )

**Receptionist:** 고객님의 의료보험카드를 복사할 수 있겠습니까?

( )

**Patient:** Sure. Here is my card.

**Receptionist:** I have a Blue Card Worldwide International Claim Form for you to fill out.

**Patient:** Alright. 제가 작성해서 가지고 오겠습니다.

( )

**Receptionist:** Thank you.

그리고 진료비 청구서와 진단서 사본이 필요하십니까?

( )

**Patient:** That's right. 만일의 경우에, 제가 고국으로 돌아가서 보험회사에 의료비를 청구하기 위해 필요한 서류들입니다.

( )

Thank you for your consideration.

## 6. Blue Card World Wide International Claim Form
블루카드 국제 의료보험 청구서 양식

- **Blue Card World Wide International Claim Form Sample,**
  **블루카드 국제 의료보험 청구서 견본**
- **Blue Card World Wide International Claim Form,**
  **블루카드 국제 의료보험 청구서 양식**
- **Drill: Let's Fill out the Blue Card International Claim Form,**
  **연습문제: 블루카드 국제 의료보험 청구서 양식 작성하기**

## Blue Card World Wide International Claim Form Sample

# BlueCard Worldwide® International Claim Form

BlueCross BlueShield

Blue Cross and Blue Shield Plans are independent licensees of the Blue Cross and Blue Shield Association.

Please see the instructions on the reverse side of this form before completing. Please type or print.
Send completed form to: BlueCard Worldwide Service Center
P.O. Box 72017
Richmond, VA 23255-2017 USA

**1. Patient Information**– 1A. Alpha prefix Identification number *Copy this from your Blue Cross Blue Shield identification card.*
XYZ 123456789

1B. Patient's name (First, middle initial, last) CHRIS A. HILL
1C. Patient's date of birth MM/DD/YYYY 03/15/1960
1D. Patient's sex ☒ Male ☐ Female
1E. Name of subscriber (First, middle initial, last) CHRIS A. HILL
1F. Subscriber's date of birth MM/DD/YYYY 03/15/1960
1G. Patient's relationship to subscriber ☒ Self ☐ Spouse ☐ Child
1H. Subscriber's current mailing address (Street, city, state, and country or ZIP code)
45 FOREST AVENUE, CHICAGO, ILLINOIS 60601 USA

**2. Other Health Insurance**– Is the patient covered under other health insurance, including Medicare A or B? ☐ Yes ☒ No
*If yes, complete 2A through 2K below.*

2A. Name and address of insuring company

2B. Type of policy ☐ Family ☐ Individual
2C. Effective date MM/DD/YYYY / /
2D. Termination date MM/DD/YYYY / /
2E. Policy or identification number of other coverage
2F. Type of coverage Hospital: ☐ Yes ☐ No Medical: ☐ Yes ☐ No Mental illness: ☐ Yes ☐ No
2G. Name of subscriber
2H. Date of birth MM/DD/YYYY / /
2I. Employer of subscriber
2J. Employment status ☐ Active employee ☐ Retired employee
2K. If patient is covered under Medicare, complete the following: Medicare Part A: ☐ Yes ☐ No Effective date ______ Medicare Part B: ☐ Yes ☐ No Effective date ______

**3. Diagnosis**– 3A. Describe illness, injury, or symptoms requiring treatment
STREP THROAT, DIFFICULTLY SWALLOWING AND FEVER
3B. Was patient's treatment due to a work-related accident or condition? ☐ Yes ☒ No

3C. Complete for care related to accidental injuries
Date of accident ______ Location: ☐ At home ☐ Auto ☐ Other ______
Time of accident ______ *If the accident was caused by someone else, attach a statement describing the accident.*

SAMPLE

**4. Charges**– Use a separate line to list each type of service or provider and attach itemized bills for all services.

| 4A. Name and address of provider making charge | 4B. Type of provider | 4C. Description of service | 4D. Dates of service or purchase | 4E. Charges |
|---|---|---|---|---|
| DR. JOHN SMITH 28 NORTH AVENUE LONDON, UK E1 4DG | PHYSICIAN (GENERAL PRACTICE) | CONSULTATION | 8/1/06 | GBP 50 |

**5. Payee**– Select one of the following payment options:
5A. ☒ Make payment to subscriber; provider has been paid.
1. Currency– Do you want the check issued in the currency reflected on the itemized bill(s) or in U.S. dollars? ☒ Currency on itemized bill(s) ☐ U.S. dollars
2. Payment Method – Do you want to receive payment via a check or bank wire? ☐ Check Provide current telephone number ______
☒ Bank Wire. If you want to receive a bank wire provide the following:
Subscriber name as it appears on bank account: CHRIS A. HILL Bank name XYZ BANK
Bank's Physical Address 100 LASALLE STREET, CHICAGO, IL 60602
Account # 12345678 ABA# ABCDEFGHIJ

5B. ☐ Make payment to provider (hospital, doctor). Please complete and sign.
Authorization for Assignment of Benefits
I, the undersigned, authorize and request Blue Cross and Blue Shield to make payment for benefits due herein to:
Name of provider ______ Signature of subscriber or spouse ______ Date ______

**6. Signature**– I certify the above is complete and correct and that I am claiming benefits only for charges incurred by the patient named above. Authorization is hereby given to any provider of service, that participated in any way in the patient's care, to release to the subscriber's Blue Cross and Blue Shield Plan and its business associates in any country any medical or other personal information that they deem necessary to provide service or adjudicate this claim, recognizing that applicable law concerning personal information may differ among countries. Authorization is also given to the subscriber's Blue Cross and Blue Shield Plan and its business associates in any country to collect, use or release any medical or other personal information that they deem necessary to provide service or adjudicate a claim.

Signature of subscriber or patient C. Hill Date 09/01/2006

## Blue Card World Wide International Claim Form

**1. Patient Information– 1A. Alpha prefix  Identification number** *Copy this from your Blue Cross Blue Shield identification card.*

| **1B. Patient's name** (First, middle initial, last) | **1C. Patient's date of birth** MM/DD/YYYY / / | **1D. Patient's sex** ☐ Male ☐ Female |
|---|---|---|
| **1E. Name of subscriber** (First, middle initial, last) | **1F. Subscriber's date of birth** MM/DD/YYYY / / | **1G. Patient's relationship to subscriber** ☐ Self ☐ Spouse ☐ Child |

**1H. Subscriber's current mailing address** (Street, city, state, and country or ZIP code)

**2. Other Health Insurance– Is the patient covered under other health insurance, including Medicare A or B?** ☐ Yes ☐ No
*If yes, complete 2A through 2K below.*

**2A. Name and address of insuring company**

| **2B. Type of policy** ☐ Family ☐ Individual | **2C. Effective date** MM/DD/YYYY / / | **2D. Termination date** MM/DD/YYYY / / | **2E. Policy or identification number of other coverage** |
|---|---|---|---|
| **2F. Type of coverage** Hospital: ☐ Yes ☐ No Medical: ☐ Yes ☐ No Mental illness: ☐ Yes ☐ No | | **2G. Name of subscriber** | **2H. Date of birth** MM/DD/YYYY / / |
| **2I. Employer of subscriber** | | | **2J. Employment status** ☐ Active employee ☐ Retired employee |

**2K. If patient is covered under Medicare, complete the following:** Medicare Part A: ☐ Yes ☐ No Effective date ______ Medicare Part B: ☐ Yes ☐ No Effective date ______

| **3. Diagnosis– 3A. Describe illness, injury, or symptoms requiring treatment** | **3B. Was patient's treatment due to a work-related accident or condition?** ☐ Yes ☐ No |
|---|---|

**3C. Complete for care related to accidental injuries**
Date of accident ______ Location: ☐ At home ☐ Auto ☐ Other ______
Time of accident ______ *If the accident was caused by someone else, attach a statement describing the accident.*

**4. Charges– Use a separate line to list each type of service or provider and attach itemized bills for all services.**

| **4A. Name and address of provider making charge** | **4B. Type of provider** | **4C. Description of service** | **4D. Dates of service or purchase** | **4E. Charges** |
|---|---|---|---|---|
| | | | | |

**5. Payee– Select one of the following payment options:**

**5A. ☐ Make payment to subscriber; provider has been paid.**
Currency– Do you want the check issued in the currency reflected on the itemized bill(s) or in U.S. dollars? ☐ Currency on itemized bill(s) ☐ U.S. dollars
Please specify subscriber name as it appears on bank account: ______

**5B. ☐ Make payment to provider (hospital, doctor).** Please complete and sign.
Authorization for Assignment of Benefits
I, the undersigned, authorize and request Blue Cross and Blue Shield to make payment for benefits due herein to:
Name of provider ______ Signature of subscriber or spouse ______ Date ______

**6. Signature–** I certify the above is complete and correct and that I am claiming benefits only for charges incurred by the patient named above. Authorization is hereby given to any provider of service, that participated in any way in the patient's care, to release to the subscriber's Blue Cross and Blue Shield Plan and its business associates in any country any medical or other personal information that they deem necessary to provide service or adjudicate this claim, recognizing that applicable law concerning personal information may differ among countries. Authorization is also given to the subscriber's Blue Cross and Blue Shield Plan and its business associates in any country to collect, use or release any medical or other personal information that they deem necessary to provide service or adjudicate a claim.

Signature of subscriber or patient ______ Date ______

위의 **Blue Card World Wide International Claim Form**을 다시 적은 것 입니다.

**1. Patient Information— 1A. Alpha prefix Identification number**

*Copy this from your Blue Cross Blue Shield identification card.*

**1B. Patient's name** (First, middle initial, last)

**1C. Patient's date of birth** MM/DD/YYYY

**1D. Patient's sex** Male____ Female____

**1E. Name of subscriber** (First, middle initial, last)

**1F. Subscriber's date of birth** MM/DD/YYYY

**1G. Patient's relationship to subscriber**

Self___ Spouse___ Child___

**1H. Subscriber's current mailing address**

(Street, city, state, and country or ZIP code)

**2. Other Health Insurance— Is the patient covered under other health insurance, including Medicare A or B?**

Yes___ No___

*If yes, complete 2A through 2K below.*

**2A. Name and address of insuring company**

**2B.Type of policy**

Family___ Individual___

**2C. Effective date** MM/DD/YYYY

**2D. Termination date** MM/DD/YYYY

**2E. Policy or identification number of other coverage**

**2F.Type of coverage**

Hospital: Yes___ No___

Medical: Yes___ No___ Mental illness: Yes___ No___

**2G. Name of subscriber**

**2H. Date of birth** MM/DD/YYYY

**2I. Employer of subscriber**

**2J. Employment status**

Active employee___ Retired employee___

**2K. If patient is covered under Medicare, complete the following:**

Medicare Part A: Yes____ No____

Effective date ___________

Medicare Part B: Yes_____ No___

Effective date ___________

**3. Diagnosis— 3A. Describe illness, injury, or symptoms requiring treatment**

**3B. Was patient's treatment due to a work-related accident or condition?**

Yes____ No____

**3C. Complete for care related to accidental injuries**

Date of accident ________________________________________

Location: At home___ Auto___ Other ______________

Time of accident ________________________________________

*If the accident was caused by someone else, attach a statement describing the accident.*

**4. Charges— Use a separate line to list each type of service or provider and attach itemized bills for all services.**

**4A. Name and address of provider making charge**

**4B. Type of provider**

**4C. Description of service**

**4D. Dates of service or purchase**

**4E. Charges**

**5. Payee— Select one of the following payment options:**

**5A. Make payment to subscriber; provider has been paid.**

Currency— Do you want the check issued in the currency reflected on the itemized bill(s) or in U.S. dollars?

Currency on itemized bill(s)_____ U.S. dollars_____

Please specify subscriber name as it appears on bank account:

_______________________________________

**5B. Make payment to provider (hospital, doctor).** Please complete and sign.

Authorization for Assignment of Benefits

I, the undersigned, authorize and request Blue Cross and Blue Shield to make payment for benefits due herein to:

Name of provider _______________________________________

Signature of subscriber or spouse _______________________________

Date ______________________

**6. Signature**— I certify the above is complete and correct and that I am claiming benefits only for charges incurred by the patient named above. Authorization is hereby given to any provider of service, that participated in any way in the patient's care, to release to the subscriber's Blue Cross and Blue Shield Plan and its business associates in any country any medical or other personal information that they deem necessary to provide service or adjudicate this claim, recognizing that applicable law concerning personal information may differ among countries. Authorization is also given to the subscriber's Blue Cross and Blue Shield Plan and its business associates in any country to collect, use or release any medical or other personal information that they deem necessary to provide service or adjudicate a claim.

Signature of subscriber or patient

______________________________________

Date ______________________

## Drill: Let's Fill out the Blue Card World Wide International Claim Form

아래의 카드를 보시고 국제의료보험양식의 1번을 작성해 보세요.

제공되지 않은 정보는 본인의 정보로 대신하세요.

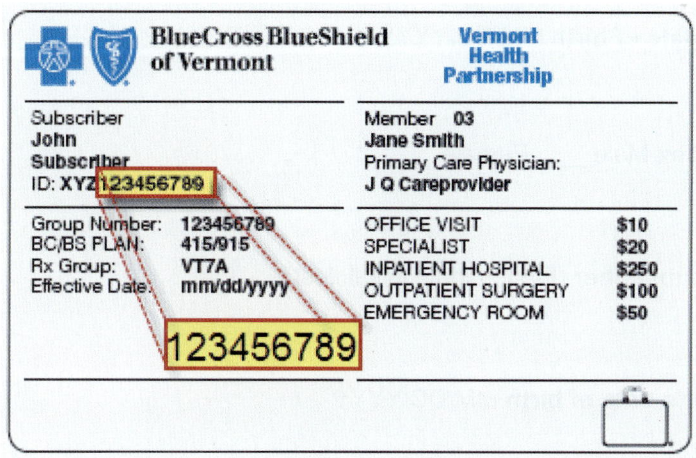


*** Jane Smith is John Subscriber's wife.**

**1. Patient Information— 1A. Alpha prefix Identification number**

*Copy this from your Blue Cross Blue Shield identification card.*

**1B. Patient's name** (First, middle initial, last)

**1C. Patient's date of birth** MM/DD/YYYY

**1D. Patient's sex** Male____ Female____

**1E. Name of subscriber** (First, middle initial, last)

**1F. Subscriber's date of birth** MM/DD/YYYY

**1G. Patient's relationship to subscriber**

Self___ Spouse___ Child___

**1H. Subscriber's current mailing address**

(Street, city, state, and country or ZIP code)

## 7. Reading Material
독해구문

- **What if I demonstrate extreme financial hardship?**
  **내가 심각한 재정난을 겪고 있다면?**

- **Words, 어휘**

### What if I demonstrate extreme financial hardship?

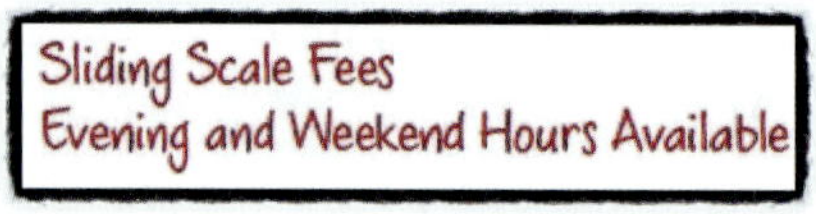


For those with extreme financial hardship, a sliding scale arrangement is available. For many individuals who suffer mental health problems, the cost of receiving proper counseling or therapy prohibits them from seeking the help that they so greatly need.

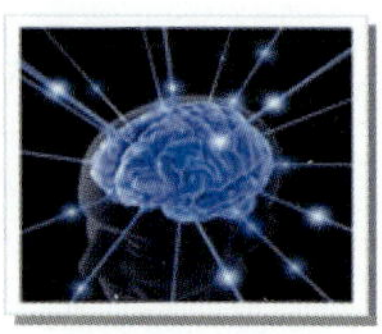

Throughout the past several decades, the cost of mental health treatment has skyrocketed, and more and more individuals suffer from lack of proper therapy. Most government-funded mental health centers and some private therapists, however, offer sliding scale fees in order to make treatment more affordable for low-income individuals or for those who have difficulty paying the full price of treatment due to other factors.

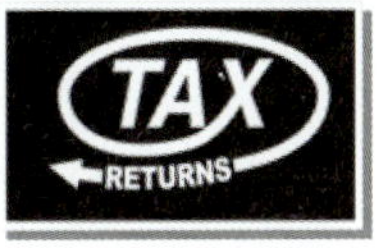


In order to qualify for a lesser fee for your treatment, you'll most likely need to fill out a detailed questionnaire as to your financial background and may perhaps need to provide documents that support your claims, such as tax returns.

Sliding scale fees are primarily based on income, although doctors will take into consideration other determining factors such as the size of your family.

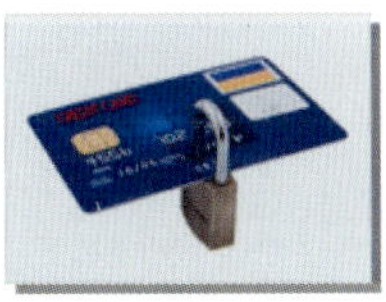

Clinics and other mental health facilities are responsible for advertising the fact that they offer a sliding scale fee and patients are encouraged to apply for it at the onset of treatment. If you cannot find notice in regards to this method of payment, it's important to ask a staff member before committing to any other payment plan. Be sure to read all the guidelines pertaining to the sliding scale fees offered by any particular facility.

**Chapter 3**

---

## Words

* financial hardship: 경제난

* sliding scale arrangement: 차등납부제

* mental health problems: 정신질환

* skyrocketed: (가격이 높이) 치솟았다

* decade: 십 년

* government-funded: 정부보조를 받는

* affordable: ~을 받을 수 있도록

* low-income: 저임금

* questionnaire: 질문서

* tax returns: 세금 환급증명서

* primarily: 기본적으로

* take into consideration: ~을 고려하다

* the onset: 시작

* regards to: ~에 관한

* committing to: ~을 결정하는 것

* pertaining to: ~의, ~에 관한

* facility: 시설

## 8. 정답 및 해석

## Chapter 3

### 1. 진료비 관련 주요어휘

#### 플라스틱 화폐란 무엇입니까?

**신용카드나 직불카드를 받습니까?**

해석: 플라스틱 화폐는 현금 또는 기존의 화폐를 대신하는 것입니다.
플라스틱 화폐는 우리가 일상생활에서 구매하기 위해 사용하는
신용카드 또는 직불카드를 말합니다

## 2. 의료보험이 없는 외국인 입원 환자의 경우

### 대화 1

**Receptionist:** 병원비를 어떻게 지불하시겠습니까? 의료보험이 있습니까?
**Patient:** 아닙니다. 제가 자비로 지불할 것입니다.

**Receptionist:** 알겠습니다. 의료보험에 가입하지 않으셨으면, 보증금을 내셔야 합니다.
**Patient:** 보증금으로 얼마를 지불해야 하나요?

**Receptionist**: 의료비의 반액을 지불하셔야 합니다.
그리고 나머지 반액은 퇴원하시는 날에 완불하셔야 합니다.
**Patient:** 알겠습니다. 신용카드도 받으시나요?

**Receptionist:** 예. 비자카드를 받습니다.
**Patient:** 그러면 비자카드로 지불하겠습니다.
그런데, 받은 혈액검사 비용은 얼마인가요?

**Receptionist:** $100.00 입니다.
**Patient:** 알겠습니다. 총 얼마를 지불해야 하나요?

**Receptionist:** 보증금과 합해서 $1,500 입니다.
**Patient:** 알겠습니다. 제 비자카드 여기 있습니다.

**Receptionist:** 예. 비자카드로 결제해 드리겠습니다.

## 3. 주요구문

### 연습문제: 정답

접수 창구는 어디에 있습니까?

Where's the registration desk, please?

접수 용지를 어디 가면 얻을 수 있을까요?

Where can I get a registration form?

그녀의 순서대기표는 17번입니다.

She has a waiting ticket number 17.

의료보험이 있습니까?

Do you have medical insurance?

Are you covered under health insurance?

Are you covered by any health insurance?

이것이 저의 의료보험증서입니다.

Here's my health insurance certificate.

의료보험 양식은 여기에 제출해야 합니까?

Do I need to submit my medical insurance form here?

한국에 오기 전에 의료보험에 가입하셨습니까?

Have you purchased medical insurance before coming to Korea?

진찰료는 얼마이지요?

What's the fee, please?

진료상담비는 얼마인가요?

How much do you charge for a consultation?

이 혈액검사 비용은 얼마입니까?

How much do you charge for the blood test?

비용은 얼마 되지 않습니다.

It won't cost much.

진료실은 어디 있어요?

Where's the doctor's examination room, please?

진료상담실은 어디 있어요?

Where's the consultation room, please?

## 4. 해외의료보험이 있는 경우

### 연습문제: 개인수표작성하기

**정답**

**Name:** Lorri Oh **117**
**Address:** # 703 Spy Glass Apt
**City, State, Zip:** Salt Lake, UT 84103

**Date:** 02/20/2011

**Pay to the**

**Order of** University of Utah Book Store $ 40.25

*Forty and 25/100* **Dollars**

**Bank Name:** Zion's Bank
**Bank Address:** 72 Main Street
Salt Lake City, UT 84109

**Memo:** Biochem text book Signature ______________

* 하단의 서명란에 본인의 사인을 하시면 됩니다.

## 진단서

### 진단서

아래에 서명한 담당의사인 (성명)................................................

본인은 홍길동의 (홍길동의 성명) 혈액검사결과와 흉부 엑스레이검사를 했음을 증명합니다.

..........................................................................................................

국적:.......................................................................................................

여권번호:..................................................................................................

출생날짜와 장소:........................................................................................

거주지:....................................................................................................

그 또는 그녀에게서 아래의 소견을 발견했습니다. (해당사항에 표시하세요):

| | 아래의 질병 소견 없음 | 아래의 질병을 앓고 있음 |
|---|---|---|
| 에이즈 | | |
| B형과 C형 간염 | | |
| 결핵 | | |
| 매독 | | |

발행기관................................................날짜...................................

의사서명...................................................................................................

병원직인...................................................................................................

## 5. 해외보험이 있는 외래환자

### 대화 2

**Receptionist:** 진료비를 어떻게 지불하시겠습니까?

**Patient:** 저는 외국 의료보험에 가입돼 있습니다. 보험처리가 가능할까요?

**Receptionist:** 의료보험회사의 이름이 무엇입니까?

**Patient:** 저는 블루크로스 블루쉴드 의료 보험에 가입되어 있습니다.

**Receptionist:** 의료보험회사로부터 의료보험 보증서를 받아오셨나요?

**Patient:** 예. 여기 있습니다.

**Receptionist:** 제가 확인하겠습니다.
제가 고객님의 보험회사와 우리병원이 직접 청구하는 방식을 따르는지 확인해 보겠습니다.

**Patient:** 알겠습니다.

**Receptionist:** 좋은 소식입니다.
고객님의 보험회사는 우리병원과 직접 청구하는 계약을 맺은 회사입니다. 하지만 고객님은 공동부담금과 같은 청구서의 일부는 지불하셔야 합니다.

**Patient:** 알겠습니다. 공동부담금을 제 신용카드로 지불해도 되나요?

**Receptionist:** 예, 지불 가능합니다.

**Patient:** 얼마인가요?

**Receptionist:** 공동부담금은 $30입니다.
**Patient:** 그러면 총 진료비는 얼마인가요?

**Receptionist:** 총 진료비는 $3,500입니다.
**Patient:** 알겠습니다.

**Receptionist:** 고객님의 의료보험에 관해 질문을 하겠습니다. 의료보험 계약번호가 무엇입니까?
**Patient:** 제 의료보험 계약번호는 ANF 255-98-2364입니다.

**Receptionist:** 보험가입자의 이름은 무엇입니까?
**Patient:** 켄 존슨입니다.

**Receptionist:** 현재 거주지의 주소는요?
**Patient:** 스파이 글라스 아파트 703호, 3rd Ave, 솔트레이크시티, 유타주입니다.

**Receptionist:** 의료보험 효력발생일은 언제부터입니까?
**Patient:** 1995년 9월 12일입니다.

**Receptionist:** 지금 고용상태는요?
**Patient:** 직장에서 근무하고 있습니다.

**Receptionist:** 고객님의 의료보험카드를 복사할 수 있겠습니까?
**Patient:** 물론입니다. 카드 여기 있습니다.

**Receptionist:** 제가 고객님께서 작성하실 블루카드 월드와이드 국제 보험청구서 양식을 드리겠습니다.

**Patient:** 알겠습니다. 제가 작성해서 가지고 오겠습니다.

**Receptionist:** 감사합니다. 그리고 진료비 청구서와 진단서 사본이 필요하십니까?

**Patient:** 네, 그렇습니다. 만일의 경우에, 제가 고국으로 돌아가서 보험회사에 의료비를 청구하기 위해 필요한 서류들입니다.
배려해 주셔서 감사합니다.

## 6. 블루카드 국제 의료보험 청구서 양식 해석

**환자정보-1A.** *블루크로스 블루쉴드 아이디카드에 적혀있는* **알파벳으로 시작하는 아이디번호를** *똑같이 적으세요.*

**1B. 환자의 이름 (이름, 중간이름의 약자, 성)**

**1C. 환자의 생년월일**

**월/일/년 / /**

**1D. 환자의 성별**

**남성____ 여성____**

**1E. 보험가입자의 성명** (이름, 가운데이름 약자, 성)

**1F. 보험가입자의 생년월일**

**월/일/년 / /**

**1G. 환자와 보험가입자와의 관계**

본인____ 배우자____ 자녀____

**1H. 보험가입자의 현주소**

(번지, 도시, 주, 국가 또는 우편번호)

**2. 다른 건강보험— 환자가 Medicare A또는 Medicare B를 비롯한 다른 건강보험에 가입되어 있나요?**

예___ 아니오___

*가입이 되었다면, 아래의 2A-2K사항을 작성하세요.*

**2A. 가입된 보험회사의 이름과 주소**

**2B. 보험종류**

가족보험____ 개인보험___

**2C. 효력발생일**

**월/일/년 / /**

**2D. 만기일**

월/일/년 / /

**2E. 다른 보험의 계약번호 또는 아이디번호**

**2F. 의료급여적용의 종류**

병원: 예____ 아니오___

의료: 예_____ 아니오_____ 정신질환: 예_____ 아니오_____

**2G. 보험가입자 이름**

**2H. 생년월일** 월/일/년

**2I. 보험가입자의 고용주 이름**

**2J. 고용상태**

현재 고용되어 있음____ 은퇴____

**2K. 만일 환자가 메디케어에 가입되어 있다면, 아래의 내용을 작성하세요:**

메디케어 A: 예___ 아니오___ 메디케어 B: 예___ 아니오___

효력발생일_____________ 효력발생일_____________

**3. 진단- 3A. 치료가 필요한 질병, 상해, 또는 증상을 설명하세요.**

**3B. 환자의 치료가 일과 관련된 사고 또는 상태로 기인한 것입니까?**

예____ 아니오__

**3C. 사고 관련 상해로 받은 치료에 대해 작성하세요.**

사고발생 일자________________________________________

장소: 집______ 교통사고_____ 기타____________

사고발생 시간________________________________________

*만일 그 사고가 타인에 의한 것이라면, 그 사고를 설명한 진술서를 첨부하세요.*

**4. 비용---각각의 진료와 의사선생님을 각각 다른 줄에 기입하고 모든 진료에 관한 개별 청구서를 첨부하세요.**

**4A. 진료비를 청구한 과목 의사의 이름과 주소**

**4B. 진료과목 의사**

**4C. 진료받은 내용**

**4D. 의료서비스를 받거나 또는 의약품을 구매한 일자**

**4E. 진료비**

**5. 보험금 수령자-다음 지불방법 중 한 가지를 선택하세요:**

**5A. 보험금을 보험 가입자에게 지불한다; 의사는 진료비를 이미 수령했다.**

통화-세부청구서에 반영된 통화로 수표를 발급받기를 원하세요 아니면 미국달러로 발급받기를 원하세요?

세부청구서에 반영된 통화____ 미국달러____

보험가입자의 이름을 은행계좌에 표시된 대로 명시하시오:

________________________________________

**5B. 의료진(병원, 의사)에게 보험금을 지불하세요**. 모든 사항을 작성하시고 서명하세요.

보험금 지불을 위한 승인

아래에 서명한 본인은 블루크로스 블루쉴드가 여기서 청구되는 보험료를 지급하도록 재가하고 요청합니다:

의사의 성명________________________________________

보험가입자 또는 배우자의 서명________________________________

일자_______________________

**서명**-본인은 위의 사항이 완전하고 올바르며 상기 환자에 의해 초래된 비용에 대해서만 보험료를 청구함을 증명합니다.

이로써 개인정보에 관련되어 적용되는 법률이 국가마다 다르다는 점을 인정하며 환자를 치료하는데 어떠한 방식으로든 참여한 모든 의료진에게 보험청구를 심사하는데 필요하다고 생각되는 모든 의학적 및 그 밖의 개인 정보를 보험가입자의 블루크로스 블루쉴드 보험 및 세계 모든 국가에 있는 거래처에 제공할 권한을 부여합니다. 또한 보험가입자의 블루크로스 블루쉴드 보험 및 세계 모든 국가에 있는 그 거래처에서 진료를 하거나 보험 청구를 심사하는데 필요하다고 생각되는 의학적 및 그 밖의 개인정보를 수집, 사용 및 공개하도록 권한이 부여됩니다.

보험가입자 또는 환자의 서명

______________________________

일자______________________

**연습문제: 블루카드 국제 의료보험 청구서 (1번) 양식작성하기**
**정답**

## Blue Card World Wide International Claim Form

**1. Patient Information— 1A. Alpha prefix Identification number**

*Copy this from your Blue Cross Blue Shield identification card.*

**XYZ 123456789**

**1B. Patient's name** (First, middle initial, last)

**Jane Smith**

**1C. Patient's date of birth** MM/DD/YYYY

**01/02/77 (본인의 생년월일을 기입하셔도 됩니다.)**

**1D. Patient's sex** Male____ Female__✓__

**1E. Name of subscriber** (First, middle initial, last)

**John Subscriber**

**1F. Subscriber's date of birth** MM/DD/YYYY

**03/04/73 (본인의 생년월일을 기입하셔도 됩니다.)**

**1G. Patient's relationship to subscriber**

Self___ Spouse_✓__ Child___

**1H. Subscriber's current mailing address**

(Street, city, state, and country or ZIP code)

**#703 Spy Glass Apt**
**SLC, UT 84103**

## 7. 독해구문

**내가 심각한 재정난을 겪고 있다면?**

심각한 경제난을 겪는 사람들은 차등납부제를 이용할 수 있습니다.
정신질환을 앓는 많은 사람들에게, 적절한 상담 또는 치료에 드는 비용으로 인해 그들이 정말 필요로 하는 도움을 청하지 못하게 됩니다.

지난 수 십 년 동안에 걸쳐, 정신질환 치료비용은 높이 치솟았고 점점 더 많은 사람들이 적절한 치료의 부재로 고통을 겪고 있습니다.
그러나, 정부보조를 받는 대부분의 정신 건강 센터와 일부 개인 치료사들은 저임금 수급자들 또는 다른 요인들로 인해 정상치료비를 지불할 수 없는 개인들이 치료를 더 쉽게 받을 수 있도록 차등 납부제를 제공합니다.

적은 진료비에 대한 자격을 갖추려면, 당신의 경제상황에 관하여 상세한 질문서를 작성해야 할 것이고 당신의 청구를 증명하기 위해 세금 환급증명서와 같은 서류를 제출해야 할 것입니다.
차등납부제는 기본적으로는 소득에 근거하나 의사들은 가족의 수와 같은 다른 요소들도 고려하여 결정합니다.

병원 또는 다른 정신건강 시설들은 차등납부제를 제공한다고 선전할 책임이 있고 환자들은 그들이 치료를 받기 시작할 때부터 차등 납부제를 신청하도록 권장됩니다.

만일 당신이 이러한 지불방법에 관한 공지를 찾을 수 없다면, 다른 지불방법을 결정하기 전에 직원에게 물어보는 것이 매우 중요합니다.
특정한 시설이 제공하는 차등납부제의 지침서를 꼭 읽어보세요

## *Reference*

University of Utah Hospital

Wikipedia

http://therapistunlimited.com

bcbsvt.com

http://www.bcbs.com/coverage/bluecard/bluecard-worldwide.html